Fibromyalgia Vegan Delights

Recipes for Health, Relief, and Rehabilitation.

Michael Murray

All rights reserved. No part of this publication may be reproduced, distributed, or transmitted in any form or by any means, including photocopying, recording, or other electronic or mechanical methods, without the prior written permission of the publisher, except in the case of brief quotations embodied in critical reviews and certain other noncommercial uses permitted by copyright law.

Copyright © Micheal Murray, 2022.

CONTENT

Chapter 1: Foundations That Are Fibromyalgia-Friendly

Chapter 2: Energy-Dense Smoothies for Optimal Morning Performance

Chapter 3: Breakfast Bowls That Are Fibro-Friendly

Chapter 4: Comforting Soups to Calm the Soul

Chapter 5: Powerful Lunch Bowls to Boost Your Midday Energy

Chapter 6: Plant-Based Proteins for the Maintenance of Muscle

Chapter 7: Appetising Dinners for Evening Refuelling

Chapter 8: Filling Snacks for a Well-Balanced Diet

Chapter 9: Sweet Gratification with Guilt-Free Desserts

Chapter 10: Smoothies and Restorative Drinks

Chapter 11: Spices and Herbs that Reduce Inflammation

Chapter 12: Techniques for Effortless Meal Preparation

Chapter 13: Integration of a Holistic Lifestyle

Chapter 14: Mild Movement and Exercise for Fibromyalgia

Chapter 15: Integration of a Holistic Lifestyle

BONUS: MEAL PLANNER

INTRODUCTION

We invite you to join us on a transformative culinary journey through the world of plant-powered gastronomy in "Fibromyalgia Vegan Delights: Recipes for Health, Relief, and Rehabilitation." Our mission is to become a beacon of hope and rejuvenation for those navigating the complex landscape of fibromyalgia, while also delighting your palate with vibrant flavours and compassionate choices.

Every dish in these chapters serves as a testimony to the remarkable potential that exists when thoughtful veganism and subtle, multifaceted fibromyalgia symptom treatment come together. We encourage you to discover a world where every meal is intentionally created to not only fulfil gourmet appetites but also to provide a holistic embrace to those seeking health, relief, and rehabilitation. Join us as we plunge into a cornucopia of brilliant colours, textures, and fragrant spices.

Dive into the rainbow of options, with everything from evening soups to morning energy elixirs, each creation a work of plant-based culinary art. These are not only recipes; rather, they are a celebration of life, meant to make your plate look beautiful and your body feel better.

The kitchen door is not where the trip ends. We share the benefits of anti-inflammatory herbs, walk you through calming drinks for a peaceful evening, and teach you mindful eating techniques that turn every meal into a time for self-care. Accept the easy stretches and workouts that go along with our meals to incorporate holistic wellbeing into your everyday lifestyle.

This is more than just a cookbook; it's a gastronomic refuge where the healing arts and the symphony of flavours collide. "Fibromyalgia Vegan Delights" urges you to enjoy life's bounty, one delicious mouthful at a time, regardless of whether you're new to plant-based eating or looking for creative solutions to manage your fibromyalgia symptoms.

Come along as we transform the culinary scene and demonstrate that eating well can be enjoyable and that each mouthful can lead to a life that is more lively, kind, and balanced. Set out on a trip that holds the promise of wonderful changes, love, and a route to health, relief, and rehabilitation.

Chapter 1: Foundations That Are Fibromyalgia-Friendly

In "Fibromyalgia Vegan Delights: Recipes for Health, Relief, and Rehabilitation," we set the stage for a journey that goes beyond simple food discovery in the first chapter. This chapter is a celebration of colourful, nutrient-dense foods, a manual for adopting a plant-powered lifestyle, and a starting point for controlling the symptoms of fibromyalgia.

Overview of Vegan Lifestyle

The trip starts with a look at the tenets of veganism and how they can affect the treatment of fibromyalgia. It's important to live a lifestyle that supports health and compassionate decision-making, not simply what you consume. We explore the advantages of eating a plant-based diet, which range from lowering inflammation to promoting general health.

Recipe : **Green Smoothie for Beginners**

Components:

- One cup of spinach

- One half banana

- Half a cup of chunky pineapple

- Half a cup of almond milk

- One-third cup chia seeds

Getting ready:

- Process spinach, almond milk, banana, and pineapple pieces until smooth.

- Add the chia seeds for extra fibre and omega-3 fatty acids.

- Pour into a glass and enjoy the deliciously refreshing flavour.

This green smoothie sets the stage for a journey focused on health and wellbeing by demonstrating the ease of use and nutritional possibilities of a vegan lifestyle.

Choosing Vegan Basics for the Wellness of Fibromyalgia

When dealing with fibromyalgia, it becomes critical to know the essentials of a vegan pantry. This section walks readers through the basic components of vegan cuisine that is suitable for those with fibromyalgia.

Recipe: **Buddha Bowl with Quinoa**

Components:

• A cup of quinoa, cooked

• One cup of mixed veggies, such as carrots, bell peppers, and broccoli

• Half a cup of roasted chickpeas

- One-fourth cup hummus

- One tablespoon of pumpkin seeds

- Tahini-lemon dressing

Getting ready:

- Layer the quinoa to form the bowl's bottom.

- Include the chickpeas and roasted veggies.

- Add a lemon-tahini dressing drizzle.

- Add hummus and pumpkin seeds on top.

This hearty Buddha Bowl demonstrates the richness and adaptability of plant-based ingredients for fibromyalgia-friendly cooking.

Plant-Based Proteins' Restorative Properties

As the chapter goes on, it becomes clear that plant-based proteins are strong friends in the fight against fibromyalgia. Our goal is to promote general health and the health of our muscles by investigating various sources of protein.

Recipe: **Curry with Sweet Potatoes and Lentils**

Components:

• One cup cooked red lentils

• Diced one sweet potato

• One 14-ounce can of coconut milk

• One chopped onion

• Two minced garlic cloves

• One tablespoon of curry powder

• Season with salt and pepper to taste

Getting ready:

• Soften the garlic and onions in a saucepan by sautéing them.

• Stir for two minutes after adding the chopped sweet potato and curry powder.

• Add the cooked lentils and coconut milk.

• Simmer the sweet potatoes until they become soft.

• Add salt and pepper for seasoning, then serve with quinoa or rice.

This aromatic curry of sweet potatoes and lentils highlights the filling and nutritious qualities of plant-based proteins.

Bright Vegetables: A Nutrient Rainbow

This section highlights the value of a colourful assortment of vegetables and highlights the nutrients and antioxidants found in a variety of plant-based components.

Recipe: **Tofu and Rainbow Stir-Fry**

Components:

• One cubed block of firm tofu

• Carrots, bell peppers, broccoli, and sliced snow peas

• TWO TABLETS SESAMOL

• Two tsp of soy sauce

• One tablespoon of maple syrup

• One teaspoon grated ginger

- Two minced garlic cloves

Getting ready:

- In sesame oil, sauté tofu till golden brown.

- Stir-fry the veggies until they are crisp-tender.

- Combine the soy sauce, maple syrup, garlic, and ginger in a small bowl.

- Drizzle stir-fry with sauce, mix to coat, and serve over brown rice.

In addition to being a palate-pleaser, this colourful stir-fry offers a variety of nutrients that promote fibromyalgia wellbeing.

In summary, a gastronomic introduction to well-being

As we get to the conclusion of the first chapter, the scene is set for a culinary adventure that combines fibromyalgia-friendly techniques with veganism. Every meal, from filling lentil and sweet potato curries to nutrient-dense green smoothies, demonstrates the delectable possibilities of a plant-based diet. Come along on this culinary adventure where, one delicious meal at a time, healing, alleviation, and rehabilitation come together.

Chapter 2: Energy-Dense Smoothies for Optimal Morning Performance

Welcome to a chapter devoted to the practice of morning vigour and renewal, where every drink is a flavour explosion, an energy boost, and an enhancement to your day. We know how important a healthy start is, which is why in "Fibromyalgia Vegan Delights," we explore the world of Power-Packed Smoothies that are meant to energise, nourish, and create a great vibe for the day.

Overview of Morning Joy Smoothies

Your day starts with the Morning Bliss Smoothie, a carefully curated blend of nutrient-dense ingredients that will invigorate your morning as the sun rises. This smoothie, which is full of vitamins, antioxidants, and plant-based deliciousness, is not just a drink; it's a daily routine that promotes general health.

Recipe: **Energizer with Berries**

Components:

- One cup of mixed berries, including raspberries, blueberries, and strawberries

- One mature banana

- 1/2 cup frozen or fresh spinach leaves

- One-third cup chia seeds

- One cup of soy, almond, or coconut milk

- Ice cubes, if desired

Getting ready:

- In a blender, combine the mixed berries, ripe banana, chia seeds, spinach leaves, and plant-based milk.

- Blend until creamy and smooth.

- Blend once more after adding ice cubes, if desired.

- Transfer into a glass, add a few berries as a garnish, and drink your way to a morning energy boost.

***Recipe*: Refresher with Tropical Sunshine**

Components:

- One cup of chunky pineapple

- Half a mango, chopped and peeled

- Half a cup of kale leaves without stems

- One-third cup flaxseeds

- One cup of coconut water

- Ice cubes, if desired

Getting ready:

- In a blender, combine the chopped mango, pineapple pieces, flaxseeds, kale leaves, and coconut water.

Blend until silky and smooth.

If you want your smoothie cold, add ice cubes and combine one more.

- Pour into a glass with a tropical design, add a piece of pineapple as a garnish, and take a trip to a paradise on a beautiful morning.

Recipe: **Revitalising Green Goddess**

Components:

- One chopped and cored green apple

- Half a cucumber, cut into slices and peel

- Slightly damp mint leaf

- One spoonful of hemp seeds

- One cup of chilled green tea

- Ice cubes, if desired

Getting ready:

- In a blender, combine the sliced cucumber, diced green apple, hemp seeds, mint leaves, and chilled green tea.

- Process the mixture until it has a smooth consistency.

- If you want a cool drink, add ice cubes and mix again.

- Transfer into a glass, top with a mint leaf, and enjoy the deliciously crisp and green flavour.

Highlighting Nutrition to Promote Fibromyalgia Health

This chapter's smoothies are all expertly made using fibromyalgia-friendly ingredients. Leafy greens supply vital vitamins, flaxseeds contribute omega-3 fatty acids, bananas offer a potassium boost, and berries offer anti-inflammatory properties. These nutrient-dense powerhouses have been carefully chosen to promote general wellbeing and give you a peaceful start to the day.

Advice on Personalisation and Modification

Smoothies are quite adaptable, so you may customise them to fit your dietary requirements and taste preferences. Try adding a scoop of plant-based protein powder for extra protein. Try out various combinations of greens, fruits, and seeds to see what works best for you. To get the appropriate consistency, change the amount of liquid.

In conclusion, Morning Routines for Sustaining Energy

While you enjoy the bright tastes of these Power-Packed Smoothies, keep in mind that this chapter is about adopting a morning routine that nourishes your body, lifts your spirits, and creates a good outlook for the day. It's not just about blending fruits. I hope you have energetic mornings and that every drink you take will lead to a day full of healing, solace, and renewal. To the delightful adventure ahead, cheers!

Chapter 3: Breakfast Bowls That Are Fibro-Friendly

Chapter 3 is a fibromyalgia-friendly culinary experience where you start the day full of nutrients and vitality. Fibro-Friendly Breakfast Bowls are more than just a breakfast; they're a carefully balanced concoction of nutrients and flavours that will fill you up and give you a boost of energy throughout the day. Let us go into the colourful realm of these healthy breakfast options, where every dish is filled with well chosen ingredients and thoughtful preparation.

Recipe: **Breakfast Bowl with Quinoa and Berries**

Components:

• A cup of quinoa, cooked

• Half a cup of mixed berries, including raspberries, blueberries, and strawberries

• One-third cup chia seeds

- One spoonful of butter made with almonds

- One tablespoon of maple syrup

- Several chopped nuts, such as almonds or walnuts

Getting ready:

- As the foundation, arrange the cooked quinoa in a bowl.

- Add a dab of almond butter, chia seeds, and mixed berries over top.

- For sweetness, drizzle with maple syrup.

- For extra crunch, scatter some chopped nuts on top as a garnish.

- Stir everything together gently and enjoy a dish full of fibre, protein, and antioxidants.

Recipe:Bowl of Banana Walnut Breakfast Bliss

Components:

- Slabbed one ripe banana.

- Half a cup cooked rolled oats

- Chopped walnuts, 1/4 cup

- One-third cup flaxseeds

- One tsp of cinnamon

- One tablespoon of coconut flakes

Getting ready:

- Prepare the rolled oats per the directions on the box.

- Line the bottom of a bowl with the cooked oats.

- Arrange chopped walnuts, flaxseeds, and banana slices in a layer.

- For taste and warmth, sprinkle with cinnamon.

- For a touch of the tropics, sprinkle some coconut flakes on top.

- Gently stir, then savour a dish that balances the crunch of walnuts with the richness of bananas.

Recipe: Avocado and Spinach Protein Bowl

Components:

- One cup of sautéed baby spinach

- Slicing half of an avocado

Half a cup of cooked quinoa.

- 1/4 cup roasted chickpeas

- One tablespoon of pumpkin seeds

- A dressing made with two tablespoons of tahini, one lemon's juice, salt, and pepper.

Getting ready:

- After baby spinach has wilted, sauté it and put it aside.

- As the foundation, arrange cooked quinoa in a bowl.

- Arrange roasted chickpeas, sliced avocado, and sautéed spinach.

For a taste explosion, drizzle with lemon-tahini dressing.

• For extra texture, sprinkle pumpkin seeds over top.

• Gently toss, and savour a breakfast full of protein to power your day.

4. Joy Bowl with blueberries and almonds

Components:

• Half a cup of blueberries

• Almonds, sliced, 1/4 cup

• Half a cup of yoghurt made with coconut milk

• Half a cup of granola

• One tablespoon agave syrup or honey

Getting ready:

• Arrange blueberries as the bottom layer in a bowl.

• Top with a big dollop of yoghurt made with coconut milk.

For crunch, mix in some granola and chopped almonds.

• For sweetness, drizzle with agave syrup or honey.

• Gently combine the ingredients to make a delightfully flavorful and textural bowl.

Recipe: **Parfait with Chia Seed Pudding**

Components:

• Two tsp full of chia seeds

• Half a cup of almond milk

- Half a tsp vanilla extract

- Freshly cut pineapple, mango, and kiwi slices

- Granola as a foundation

Getting ready:

- Combine almond milk, vanilla essence, and chia seeds in a container.

- To make a custard, give it a good stir and refrigerate for the whole night.

- Arrange the granola and fresh fruit pieces on top of the chia seed pudding in the morning.

Layers should be repeated until the jar is full.

- Savour a parfait that's high in fibre, natural sweetness, and omega-3 fatty acids.

Final Thought: A Fulfilling Start

These Fibro-Friendly Breakfast Bowls provide a nutritional symphony that supports those managing fibromyalgia, elevating them above the ordinary. Every bowl, from the velvety Banana Walnut Bliss to the protein-rich Quinoa Berry Bowl, is an explosion of taste and nutrition. Make a conscious start to your day and use these breakfast bowls as the foundation for your path to recovery, alleviation, and well-being.

Chapter 4: Comforting Soups to Calm the Soul

The warmth and nutrition of a hot cup of soup are fundamental to the administration of fibromyalgia. The fourth chapter of

"Fibromyalgia Vegan Delights" presents a culinary paradise that leads you through a selection of comforting soups that are carefully prepared to provide you not only warmth and cosiness but also essential nutrients for your overall health.

Overview: The Curative Power of Soups

Recognising the healing potential of a cup of soup is crucial as we begin this chapter. Beyond its delicious tastes, soup is a mild healer, providing warmth to aching muscles and an abundance of nutrients to promote general well-being. With the introduction of soups that serve as both a physical haven and a spiritual solace, this chapter aims to highlight the relationship between flavour and health.

Recipe: Soup with Turmeric Lentils

Components:

- One cup of red lentils, dry

- One finely chopped onion

- Two diced carrots

- Two chopped celery stalks

- Three minced garlic cloves

- One tsp finely ground turmeric

- One teaspoon of cumin powder

- Half a teaspoon of coriander powder

- Six cups broth made with vegetables

- Season with salt and pepper to taste

- Fresh cilantro for decorating

Getting ready:

- Give lentils a quick rinse in cold water and reserve.

- Saute the celery, carrots, onions, and garlic in a big saucepan until they are tender.

- To coat the veggies, add the coriander, cumin, and turmeric and stir.

- Add the lentils and pour in the vegetable broth. After bringing to a boil, lower the heat, and cook the lentils until they are soft.

- Add pepper and salt according to taste.

- Before serving, garnish with fresh cilantro.

This lentil soup with turmeric infusion warms your body and highlights turmeric's anti-inflammatory properties, making it a reassuring ally against the symptoms of fibromyalgia.

Recipe**: Roasted Butternut Squash Soup with Creaminess**

Components:

• One medium butternut squash, diced after peeling

• One chopped onion

• Two sliced carrots

• Three minced garlic cloves

• Four cups broth made with vegetables

• A teaspoon of sage, dried

• One-half tsp nutmeg

• Season with salt and pepper to taste

• Half a cup of coconut milk, if desired

- As a garnish, pumpkin seeds

Getting ready:

- Roast garlic, carrots, onions, and butternut squash in the oven until they are soft and beginning to caramelise.

- Place the roasted veggies in a saucepan and season with salt, pepper, nutmeg, sage, and vegetable broth.

Simmer the mixture until the flavours combine.

- Process until smooth, adding coconut milk if required to make it creamier.

- Taste and adjust the spice. Garnish with pumpkin seeds and serve.

The earthy sweetness of squash and the fragrant sage combine to create a velvety butternut squash soup that is both rich and comforting, all while following fibromyalgia-friendly dietary guidelines.

Recognising the Components of Healing Soups

When making soups that are suitable for those with fibromyalgia, using the right components is essential. In-depth information on the nutritional characteristics of each component is included in Chapter 4, which helps readers make decisions that will promote their comfort and health.

Example3: Foundations of Healing Broth

• Broth made with vegetables:

• The foundation of many soups that are good for fibromyalgia is a handmade vegetable broth, which is rich in vitamins and minerals. It offers a wholesome foundation devoid of the possible inflammatory elements sometimes connected to animal broths.

• Spices that Reduce Inflammation:

• In addition to adding rich flavours to your soups, turmeric, ginger, and garlic all have anti-inflammatory effects. These spices help to reduce inflammation in the body, which helps to manage the symptoms of fibromyalgia.

• High-Nutrient Lentils:

• Iron, fibre, and plant-based protein are all abundant in lentils. They provide a nutritious boost for long-lasting energy and add to the heartiness of soups.

Useful Advice for Preparing Soup

Beyond only recipes, the chapter provides helpful advice on how to make preparing soup easy and pleasurable. These time-saving batch cooking methods and effective chopping procedures enable people to include healing soups into their routine without experiencing unnecessary stress.

***Recipe*: Convenient Batch Cooking**

Base for Golden Vegetable Soup:

• Components:

• A variety of veggies, including zucchini, sweet potatoes and carrots

• Garlic and onions for taste

• Black pepper, cumin, and turmeric have anti-inflammatory properties

• Getting ready:

• Until caramelised, roast or sauté veggies with seasonings.

- Blend to create a creamy soup base.

- Divide and freeze to make it simple and fast to use in a variety of soup recipes.

Making a flexible soup foundation ahead of time allows people to expedite their cooking routine and guarantee a warm bowl of nourishment is constantly accessible.

In summary, a harmonious blend of cosiness and sustenance

"Fibromyalgia Vegan Delights" invites readers to relish the restorative powers inherent in each expertly prepared soup as Chapter 4 develops as a symphony of solace and nutrition. These dishes capture the spirit of healing through food, from the warming anti-inflammatory qualities of turmeric lentil soup to the rich, creamy texture of roasted butternut squash soup. As the scents emanate from your kitchen, may every mouthful represent a stride towards well-being, alleviation, and recovery.

Chapter 5: Powerful Lunch Bowls to Boost Your Midday Energy

"Energising Lunch Bowls for Midday Stamina" takes centre stage in

"Fibromyalgia Vegan Delights: Recipes for Health, Relief, and Rehabilitation." This chapter is a culinary oasis, offering a collection of nutrient-packed lunch bowls designed to fuel your body, support mental focus, and manage fibromyalgia symptoms with a burst of plant-powered energy. During the middle of the day, when energy levels often dip and the need for sustained vitality is crucial, "Energising Lunch Bowls for Midday Stamina" will take centre stage.

An Overview of Midday Snacking

Lunchtime meals are essential for maintaining an even energy level and warding off exhaustion, particularly for those with fibromyalgia. This chapter begins with an examination of the dietary components that support midday energy, highlighting the need of well-balanced meals full of healthful plant-based foods.

Highlighted Ingredient: Quinoa

Quinoa is a star ingredient in our lunch bowls since it's a complete protein. Rich in vital amino acids and offering a long-lasting energy burst, it's a perfect starting point for midday meals.

Recipe: **Power Bowl of Quinoa**

Components:

- A cup of quinoa, cooked

- One cup of mixed greens (kale, spinach)

- Half a cup of cherry tomatoes

- Half a cup diced cucumber

- 1/4 cup chopped red bell pepper

- Carrots, 1/4 cup, shredded

- 1/4 cup roasted chickpeas

- Two tsp full of pumpkin seeds

- Dressing with tahini

Dressing with Tahini:

- Two tahini teaspoons

- One tsp lemon juice

- Finely chopped garlic clove

- Season with salt and pepper to taste

Getting ready:

- Combine the cooked quinoa, roasted chickpeas, cucumber, cherry tomatoes, red bell pepper, shredded carrots, and mixed greens in a bowl.

• To make the dressing, combine the tahini, lemon juice, chopped garlic, salt, and pepper in a separate small bowl.

• Top the bowl with pumpkin seeds and drizzle with tahini dressing.

• Gently toss to mix, making sure all of the ingredients are covered with the delicious dressing.

• Serve right away and savour the nutritious, protein-rich deliciousness of this vibrant quinoa meal.

Recipe: **Bowl of Chickpea and Avocado Salad**

Components:

• One cup of cooked lentils

• Diced one avocado

- One cup of mixed greens (watercress, rocket)

- Half a cup of cherry tomatoes

- 1/4 cup finely chopped red onion

- 1/4 cup diced cucumber

- Two tsp full of sunflower seeds

- Tahini-lemon dressing

Tahini-Lemon Dressing:

- Three tsp tahini

- Half a tablespoon of lemon juice

- One tablespoon of extra virgin olive oil

- One tsp of pure maple syrup

- Season with salt and pepper to taste

Getting ready:

- Put cooked chickpeas, chopped avocado, mixed greens, cherry tomatoes, red onion, and cucumber in a big bowl.

- To make the dressing, combine the tahini, lemon juice, olive oil, maple syrup, salt, and pepper in a small bowl.

Over the salad dish, drizzle the lemon-tahini dressing.

For an extra crunch, sprinkle some sunflower seeds on top.

- Gently mix the ingredients to ensure that they are uniformly coated with dressing.

- Savour the deliciousness of this nutrient-dense, refreshing chickpea avocado salad dish.

Nutritional Perspectives and Advantages

Every ingredient in these lunch bowls supports a diet that is beneficial to fibromyalgia. The mix of plant-based proteins, healthy fats, and a variety of vitamins and minerals promotes general wellbeing, while the high fibre level helps with digestion.

Recipe Ideas to Maximise Productivity

Understanding the value of efficiency in the kitchen, this chapter offers recipes that simplify the process of preparing ingredients. Some of these ideas include roasting more chickpeas for many meals, preparing vegetables for the week, and batch-cooking quinoa.

In summary, a midday symphony of tastes

Enjoying the bright colours and variety of tastes of these energetic lunch bowls can help you to fuel your body, increase your energy, and help manage the symptoms of fibromyalgia. This chapter is an invitation to turn your noon meal into a beautiful symphony of plant-powered pleasures, turning it into a healthy, relieving, and revitalising moment.

Chapter 6: Plant-Based Proteins for the Maintenance of Muscle

Chapter 6 is a powerful crescendo in the symphony of managing fibromyalgia. It presents a variety of satisfying and healthy plant-based protein meals that are designed to build muscle, aid in recovery, and add flavour to the table. As we explore the world of "Plant-Based Proteins for Muscle Support," let every recipe serve as a tribute to the harmonious union of taste, health, and nutrition.

Recipe: **Stir-fried Savoury Tempeh**

Components:

• One cubed chunk of tempeh

• Sliced mixed veggies (carrots, broccoli, and bell peppers).

• Two minced garlic cloves

• One tablespoon of soy sauce

- TWO TABLETS SESAMOL

- One teaspoon grated ginger

- Quinoa or brown rice (to serve)

Getting ready:

- Heat the sesame oil in a wok or big pan over medium-high heat.

- Add the grated ginger and minced garlic, and sauté until aromatic.

- Stir-fry the tempeh cubes until they get golden brown.

- Add a variety of colourful sliced veggies and stir-fry them until they are vibrantly tender.

- To ensure that the flavours are distributed evenly, drizzle soy sauce over the mixture.

This flavorful stir-fry is a great way to serve quinoa or brown rice for a high-protein, fibromyalgia-friendly dinner.

Recipe: Power Bowl with Lentils and Spinach

Components:

- One cup of brown or green lentils, cooked

- Newly harvested spinach

- Halved cherry tomatoes

- Diced one cucumber

- 1/4 cup coarsely chopped red onion

- Dressing with balsamic vinaigrette

Getting ready:

- Prepare lentils per the directions on the box, then set aside to cool.

- Place lentils, chopped red onion, sliced cucumber, half cherry tomatoes, and fresh spinach leaves in a bowl.

Add a balsamic vinaigrette dressing drizzle and mix until well covered.

Savour this nutrient-dense power bowl full of vital vitamins and plant-based proteins.

Recipe: **Curry with Sweet Potatoes and Chickpeas**

Components:

- One can (15 ounces) of rinsed and drained chickpeas

- Diced and peeled two medium sweet potatoes

- One 14-ounce can of coconut milk

- One finely chopped onion

- Three minced garlic cloves

- One tablespoon of curry powder

- Fresh cilantro for decoration

- Basmati (serving) rice

Getting ready:

- Until softened, sauté minced garlic and chopped onion in a big saucepan.

- Stir to coat in the fragrant base after adding the chopped sweet potatoes and chickpeas to the saucepan.

- To ensure that the flavours are distributed evenly, sprinkle curry powder on top of the mixture.

• Add the coconut milk and cook the curry for a little while.

• Simmer until the sweet potatoes are soft.

• Top this curry with sweet potatoes and chickpeas with a bed of basmati rice and some fresh cilantro for decoration.

Recipe: **Quinoa Pilaf with Grilled Tofu Skewers**

Components:

• Pressed and sliced firm tofu

• Chopped bell peppers in various combinations

• Diced red onion into wedges

• Tomatillos

- For marinating, olive oil

- Juice from lemons

- Cooked quinoa

- Parsley, fresh (for garnish)

Getting ready:

- Tofu cubes, cherry tomatoes, bell pepper pieces, and red onion wedges should all be marinated in a solution of olive oil and lemon juice.

- To make vibrant tofu skewers, thread the marinated ingredients onto skewers.

- Grill the skewers until the veggies are soft and the tofu is browned.

Serve this visually beautiful and high-protein meal over cooked quinoa sprinkled with fresh parsley.

Plant-Based Proteins: A Harmony of Nutrients

This chapter's recipes are all composed of plant-based proteins that harmonise with a wide range of tastes and textures. These recipes, which range from the hearty tempeh stir-fry to the colourful lentil and spinach power bowl, include a varied range of nutrients that are essential for maintaining healthy muscles and general wellbeing.

Ingredients Packed with Protein:

• Tempeh: Packed with of protein and probiotics, tempeh is a firm-textured, nutty-flavored fermented soy food.

• Lentils: Packed with vital minerals, fibre, and protein, lentils are a heart-healthy and adaptable option.

• Chickpeas: Rich in protein, fibre, and antioxidants, chickpeas assist healthy digestion and muscles.

• Tofu: A flexible soy-based protein source, tofu takes on the tastes of the food it is cooked with.

Enjoy the delicious confluence of health and culinary creativity with every taste of these plant-based protein treats. Let each bite be a step towards feeding your body and supporting the health of your muscles. Greetings from the trip of plant-based proteins for supporting muscle mass—a dish full of health harmony.

Chapter 7: Appetising Dinners for Evening Refuelling

The need for a hearty and filling meal increases as the day winds down and nighttime draws near. In this section of "Fibromyalgia Vegan Delights," we look at a variety of delicious meals that are meant to soothe and accommodate fibromyalgia sufferers in addition to providing physical nourishment. Every recipe is made with a carefully balanced combination of plant-based components, chosen to meet the specific requirements of those who are managing their fibromyalgia symptoms.

Recipe: **Stuffed peppers with quinoa and roasted vegetables**

Components:

• Four big bell peppers, any hue

• One cup cooked quinoa

• One diced zucchini

- Half a cup of cherry tomatoes

- One cup of sliced mushrooms

- Half a cup of finely chopped red onion

- Two minced garlic cloves

- A single cup of tomato sauce

- One teaspoon of oregano, dried

- Season with salt and pepper to taste

- As a garnish, fresh parsley

Getting ready:

- Set oven temperature to 375°F, or 190°C.

- Slice off the bell peppers' tops, then remove the seeds and membranes.

- Put the cooked quinoa, dried oregano, dried onions, garlic, cherry tomatoes, mushrooms, zucchini and salt and pepper in a bowl.

- Stuff the quinoa mixture inside each bell pepper and put them on a baking tray.

- Cover the filled peppers with tomato sauce.

- Bake peppers for 30 to 35 minutes, or until they are soft.

- Before serving, garnish with fresh parsley.

Recipe: **Brown rice with lentil and vegetable curry**

Components:

- One cup cooked brown lentils

- One cup florets of broccoli

- One sliced carrot

- One sliced bell pepper, any colour

- One 15-ounce can of coconut milk

- Two tablespoons pasted red curry.

- One tablespoon of soy sauce

- One tablespoon of maple syrup

- One tablespoon of extra virgin olive oil

- Two minced garlic cloves

- One teaspoon grated ginger

- Brown rice cooked and ready to serve

Getting ready:

- Heat the olive oil in a big pan over medium heat.

• When aromatic, add the garlic and ginger and sauté for one to two minutes.

• Add the soy sauce, maple syrup, coconut milk, and red curry paste.

• Include the bell pepper, broccoli, carrot, and cooked lentils.

• Simmer the veggies for 15 to 20 minutes, or until they are soft.

• Toss with warm brown rice.

Recipe: Quinoa Pilaf with Grilled Tofu Skewers

Components:

• One block of pressed and diced extra-firm tofu

• One sliced courgette

- One red onion, sliced into pieces

- One bell pepper, chopped into bits, any colour

- Two teaspoons of olive oil

- Two tsp balsamic vinegar

- A teaspoon of thyme, dried

- Season with salt and pepper to taste

Quinoa Pilaf:

- One cup cooked quinoa

- 1/4 cup roasted pine nuts

- 1/4 cup finely chopped fresh parsley

- Juiced one lemon

• Season with salt and pepper to taste

Getting ready:

• Combine olive oil, salt, pepper, dried thyme, and balsamic vinegar in a basin.

• Thread red pepper, red onion, zucchini and chunks of tofu onto skewers.

• Apply marinade on skewers and cook for ten to fifteen minutes, rotating them often.

• To prepare the pilaf, combine the cooked quinoa, parsley, pine nuts, lemon juice, salt, and pepper in a separate dish.

• Top quinoa pilaf with grilled tofu skewers.

Recipe: **Steamed asparagus with baked lemon herb tilapia**

Components:

- Four fillets of tilapia

- One sliced lemon

- Two teaspoons of olive oil

- A teaspoon of thyme, dried

- One tsp of dehydrated rosemary

- Season with salt and pepper to taste

- Spears of fresh asparagus

Getting ready:

- Set oven temperature to 375°F, or 190°C.

- Arrange the fillets of tilapia on a baking pan.

- Season the fillets with salt, pepper, dried thyme, and dried rosemary after drizzling them with olive oil.

Place slices of lemon on top of each fillet.

• Bake the fish for 15 to 20 minutes, or until it is well done.

Steam asparagus in a steamer basket until it becomes soft.

• Place steamed asparagus on a bed of tilapia fillets.

These meal dishes are carefully chosen based on their ability to support fibromyalgia-friendly dietary guidelines in addition to their delicious flavours. These vegan treats put an emphasis on healthful ingredients, sumptuous textures, and alluring scents to create evening dinners that provide happiness, cosiness, and overall wellbeing.

Chapter 8: Filling Snacks for a Well-Balanced Diet

Chapter 8 welcomes you to the world of Satisfying Snacks, a variety of vegan treats that will not only satisfy your desires but also give you with well-balanced nutrients that will work in harmony with your path towards wellness. These snacks are designed to be allies in your pursuit of recovery, alleviation, and well-being—they are more than just tasty treats.

Recipe: **Bites of sweet potato hummus**

Components:

• One medium sweet potato, cut into dice and peel

• One can (15 ounces) of rinsed and drained chickpeas

• Two minced garlic cloves

• Three tsp tahini

• Two teaspoons of olive oil

- One lemon's juice

- One teaspoon of cumin powder

- Season with salt and pepper to taste

- Cucumber slices or whole grain crackers for serving

Getting ready:

- Boil or steam the sweet potato until it becomes soft.

- Put the sweet potato, chickpeas, garlic, tahini, olive oil, lemon juice, cumin, salt, and pepper in a food processor.

- Blend until smooth, stopping occasionally to scrape down the sides.

- Taste and adjust the seasoning.

Serve the sweet potato hummus as a cool, fibromyalgia-friendly snack over sliced cucumber or whole grain crackers.

***Recipe*: Rice Cakes with Avocado and Tomato**

Components:

• Cakes made with brown rice.

• One mashed, ripe avocado

• Halved cherry tomatoes

• Newly harvested basil leaves

• A balsamic glaze drizzle

• A dash of sea salt

Getting ready:

- Top each rice cake with a thick layer of mashed avocado.

- Garnish with fresh basil leaves and halved cherry tomatoes.

- Top with a little sea salt and a drizzle of balsamic glaze.

Savour these open-faced treats, which are full of fresh flavours and healthy fats, as a light and filling snack.

Recipe: **Energy Bites with Nuts**

Components:

- One cup of rolled oats

- Half a cup of almond butter

- One-fourth cup maple syrup

- 1/4 cup of flaxseed meal

- 1/4 cup chopped nuts, such walnuts or almonds

- One-fourth cup dark chocolate chips

- One tsp vanilla essence

- A dash of salt

Getting ready:

- Combine ground flaxseed, chopped almonds, chocolate chips, almond butter, maple syrup, rolled oats, vanilla essence, and a dash of salt in a big bowl.

- Mix the ingredients well by stirring.

To make handling simpler, place it in the refrigerator for half an hour.

- Form the mixture into balls that are bite-sized.

- Toss these nutty energy bits into the fridge for a simple, high-energy snack any time of the week.

Crispy Roasted Chickpeas, as an Example

Components:

- One can (15 ounces) of rinsed and drained chickpeas

- One tablespoon of extra virgin olive oil

- One tsp well-smoked paprika

- Half a teaspoon of cumin

- One-half tsp powdered garlic

- Season with salt and pepper to taste

Getting ready:

Start the oven to 400°F, or 200°C.

Using a paper towel, pat the chickpeas dry to eliminate any remaining moisture.

• Combine the chickpeas, salt, pepper, cumin, smoked paprika, and olive oil in a bowl.

• Arrange the chickpeas in a single layer on a baking sheet.

• Roast for 25 to 30 minutes, shaking the pan halfway through, or until crispy.

• Let cool completely before enjoying these roasted chickpeas, which are full of flavour and fibre.

Recipe: **Vegan Cream Cheese with Herbed Cucumber Roll-Ups**

Components:

- One cucumber, cut lengthwise into thin slices

- Cream cheese made without dairy

- Diced fresh dill

- Finely chopped chives

- Season with salt and pepper to taste

Getting ready:

- After laying the cucumber slices flat, cover each one with a thin coating of vegan cream cheese.

- Top with finely chopped chives and fresh dill.

- Add pepper and salt according to taste.

- Use toothpicks to secure the cucumber slices as you roll them up.

- With a blast of herbal deliciousness, these light and refreshing roll-ups make a great snack.

This chapter explains how snacks, which are made with components that are favourable to fibromyalgia, may be used as bridges to regulating hunger, maintaining energy levels, and loving your body. These dishes are not only tasty, but they are also designed to make you feel good and support you on your path to recovery, alleviation, and well-being.

Chapter 9: Sweet Gratification with Guilt-Free Desserts

It is not necessary to give up dessert in order to live a fibromyalgia-friendly lifestyle. This chapter explores the technique of creating decadent, guilt-free sweet delights that adhere to veganism's core values and meet the nutritional requirements of those managing fibromyalgia symptoms. Get ready for a pleasant voyage in which every dessert is a celebration of taste, sweetness, and overall health.

Recipe: **Chocolate Mousse with Avocado**

Components:

• A pair of mature avocados

• One-fourth cup cocoa powder

• One-fourth cup maple syrup

• One tsp vanilla essence

• A dash of sea salt

- Ripe berries for garnish

Getting ready:

- After removing the pit and peeling the avocados, put the flesh in a food processor or blender.

- Include vanilla essence, cocoa powder, maple syrup, and a little amount of sea salt.

- Blend, scraping down the sides as necessary, until smooth and creamy.

After transferring the mousse into serving glasses, chill it for a minimum of two hours.

- For a rich and wholesome dessert, top with fresh berries just before serving.

This avocado chocolate mousse delivers a healthy dose of antioxidants and lipids while still satisfying desires for sweets.

Recipe: Chia Pudding Parfait with Berries

Components:

4.25 oz of chia seeds

• One cup of soy, almond, or coconut milk

• One tablespoon of maple syrup

• One tsp vanilla essence

• Strawberries, blueberries, and raspberries are mixed berries.

• Granola as a foundation

Getting ready:

• Combine the plant-based milk, vanilla essence, maple syrup, and chia seeds in a bowl.

• Give it a good stir, then cover and refrigerate for at least 4 hours or overnight to enable the chia seeds absorb the liquid and become thick like pudding.

• Arrange granola and mixed berries on top of the chia pudding in serving cups.

• Continue layering and put more berries on top.

• For a cool, high-fiber dessert parfait, serve chilled.

In addition to being delicious, this berry chia pudding parfait provides a healthy balance of antioxidants and omega-3 fatty acids.

Recipe: Energy Bites with Coconut-Lime

Components:

- One cup of raw, shredded coconut

- Half a cup of finely chopped almonds

- 1/4 cup melted coconut oil

- Two tsp pure maple syrup

- One lime, zest and juice

- A dash of salt

Getting ready:

- Place crushed almonds, shredded coconut, maple syrup, melted coconut oil, lime zest, lime juice, and a dash of salt in a bowl.

- Mix until the mixture holds together and is well mixed.

- Roll the ingredients into little energy bite-sized balls with your palms.

• Transfer the coconut-lime energy bites to a tray lined with parchment paper, then chill for a minimum of half an hour.

• Savour these revitalising and refreshing nibbles as a guilt-free snack or dessert.

These coconut-lime energy bites have a zesty taste and healthy fats with a touch of tropics.

Recipe: **Crisp Baked Apples**

Components:

• Four peeled and sliced apples

• One tsp lemon juice

• One-fourth cup maple syrup

• One tsp finely ground cinnamon

Half a cup of rolled oats

• One-fourth cup almond flour

• Two teaspoons of melted coconut oil

• If desired, chopped nuts for the topping

Getting ready:

• Set oven temperature to 175°C/350°F.

• Combine the ground cinnamon, maple syrup, and lemon juice with the cut apples in a bowl.

• To make the crispy topping, combine rolled oats, almond flour, and melted coconut oil in a another bowl.

• Transfer the apple mixture to a baking dish and top with the crisp topping, distributing it evenly.

- Bake for 30 to 35 minutes, or until the apples are soft and the topping is golden brown.

- Before serving, let the cooked apple crisp cool a little. If desired, sprinkle chopped nuts on top.

This baked apple crisp combines healthful components that are appropriate for a fibromyalgia-friendly diet with the comforting flavours of a traditional dessert.

Recipe: **Nice Cream with Pumpkin Spice**

Components:

- Two ripe bananas, cut into slices, frozen

- Half a cup of pureed canned pumpkin

- One-fourth cup coconut milk

- Two tsp pure maple syrup

- One tsp pumpkin spice mixture

Getting ready:

- Place frozen banana slices, pumpkin puree, coconut milk, maple syrup, and pumpkin spice mix in a food processor or blender.

- Blend, scraping down the sides as necessary, until smooth and creamy.

- After transferring the lovely cream with pumpkin spice to a container, freeze it for a minimum of two hours.

- For a guilt-free dessert, scoop and serve this rich, autumn-inspired lovely cream.

With the additional advantages of potassium and fibre from bananas, this pumpkin spice lovely cream is a wonderful alternative to regular ice cream that perfectly captures the flavour of autumn.

Within the domain of "Fibromyalgia Vegan Delights," these guilt-free confections are more than simply culinary works of art; they are a harmonious blend of tastes intended to provide happiness, sweetness, and dietary reinforcement to anyone adopting a fibromyalgia-friendly way of living. Savour these delicious delicacies without sacrificing your health in the process.

Chapter 10: Smoothies and Restorative Drinks

When it comes to managing fibromyalgia, staying hydrated turns into a powerful remedy, and using smoothies and other restorative drinks wisely becomes essential for general wellbeing. This chapter offers you the chance to delve into a variety of calming and invigorating beverage alternatives that have been painstakingly created to reduce discomfort, nourish your body, and further your path to holistic health.

Recipe:Latte with Golden Elixir

Components:

• One cup almond milk

• One teaspoon of turmeric

• Half a teaspoon of ginger

• One-fourth teaspoon of cinnamon

• A little dash of pepper

• One teaspoon (optional) maple syrup

Getting ready:

• Bring almond milk to a simmer in a saucepan.

• Add the black pepper, cinnamon, ginger, and turmeric and whisk.

• If desired, use maple syrup to sweeten.

• Transfer into your preferred cup, enjoy the amber warmth, and let the anti-inflammatory characteristics to do their job.

Recipe: **Joyful Berry Smoothie**

Components:

- One cup of mixed berries, including raspberries, blueberries, and strawberries

- Just one banana

- One cup of spinach leaves

- Half a cup of almond milk

- One tablespoon of chia seeds

Getting ready:

- Process spinach, almond milk, banana, and berries in a blender until smooth.

- Add the chia seeds for extra fibre and omega-3 fatty acids.

- Transfer into a glass and enjoy the vivid colours and crisp flavour.

Recipe: Chamomile and Lavender Tea

Components:

• One bag of chamomile tea

Dried lavender buds, 1 tsp

• One teaspoon honey, if desired

Getting ready:

• Steep dried lavender buds and a chamomile tea bag in boiling water.

• Give the tea five minutes to absorb the soothing scent.

• If desired, sweeten with honey.

• Take a long sip and enjoy a peaceful moment as you breathe in the comforting aroma.

Recipe: **Cucumber Mint Infusion for Cooling**

Components:

- Half a cucumber, cut thinly

- Slightly damp mint leaf

- One finely sliced lemon

- One water litre

- Cubes of ice

Getting ready:

- In a pitcher, mix cucumber, mint, and lemon segments.

- Cover the ingredients with water and chill for a minimum of two hours.

- For a cool and hydrating infusion, serve over ice.

Recipe: **Anti-Inflammatory Tea with Turmeric and Ginger**

Components:

• A sliced 1-inch ginger root

One teaspoon of ground turmeric

• One tablespoon honey

• Juiced one lemon

• Two cups of water

Getting ready:

Ginger slices are added to boiling water.

• After adding the ground turmeric, simmer for ten minutes.

• Strain the liquid and stir in the lemon juice and honey.

- Take a long sip and let the warmth comfort and calm you.

Recipe: **Green Smoothie Packed with Protein**

Components:

- One cup of stem-free kale leaves

- Half a cup of chunky pineapple

- One half banana

- One scoop of powdered plant-based protein

- One cup of coconut water

Getting ready:

- Process kale, protein powder, banana, pineapple, and coconut water in a blender until smooth.

- Pour into a glass to give your day a nutrient-rich boost.

Recipe: **Citrus Rosemary Refresher**

Components:

- Two fresh rosemary sprigs

- One sliced orange

- One sliced lemon

- One-liter sparkling water

- Cubes of ice

Getting ready:

- In a pitcher, muddle one rosemary herb.

- Include lemon and orange slices.

- Add ice cubes to the mixture after dousing it with sparkling water.

- Savour the herbal and tangy beverage.

Recipe: Bowl of Tropical Turmeric Smoothie

Components:

- One cup of chunky frozen mango

- Half a cup of chunky pineapple

- Just one banana

- 1 teaspoon ground turmeric

- Blending coconut milk

Add-ons:

- Granola

- Sunflower seeds

- Coconut shreds

Getting ready:

Mango, pineapple, banana, coconut milk, turmeric, and blend until smooth.

For a tropical treat, transfer into a dish and garnish with granola, chia seeds, and shredded coconut.

***Recipe* :Matcha Latte with Mint**

Components:

- 1 teaspoon powdered matcha

- One cup almond milk

- Tobacco 1 tablespoon

- New mint leaves for decoration

Getting ready:

- Until frothy, whisk matcha powder into almond milk.

- Use maple syrup to make sweets.

- Add some fresh mint leaves as a garnish for a tasty, antioxidant-rich drink.

Recipe: Wet Aloe Vera Cooler Hydration

Components:

- One cup of coconut water

- Tbsp of aloe vera gel

- Teaspoonful of fresh lime juice

- One teaspoon honey, if desired

- Cubes of ice

Getting ready:

- Using a blender, thoroughly blend aloe vera gel, lime juice, honey, and coconut water.

- Pour over ice for a refreshing and calming drink.

Each dish in this exploration of healing drinks and smoothies is more than simply a drink; it's a sip of recovery, a dash of solace, and a gulp of energy. These fibromyalgia-friendly recipes will help you stay hydrated and will revitalise your body and mind.

Chapter 11: Spices and Herbs that Reduce Inflammation

Welcome to a world where the healing power of nature blends with the spirit of culinary talent. A symphony of flavours and scents, Chapter 11 shows you how to use anti-inflammatory herbs and spices to improve your meals and help manage the symptoms of fibromyalgia. This chapter is a herbal wonderland, full of relaxing teas and golden-hued curries that will entice you to discover the medicinal possibilities hidden in your spice cabinet.

*Recipe:*Ginger-Golden Milk with Turmeric:

Components:

• One cup soy, coconut, or almond milk made from plants

• One tsp finely ground turmeric

• One-half tsp ground ginger

- One tablespoon agave nectar or maple syrup

- A pinch of black pepper (improves absorption of turmeric)

- For added warmth, a dash of cinnamon is optional.

Getting ready:

- Heat the plant-based milk in a small saucepan over medium heat.

- Add the ginger, turmeric, black pepper, and your preferred sweetener and whisk.

Stirring constantly, heat the mixture until it's hot but not boiling.

- Transfer into a cup, garnish with cinnamon if like, and enjoy the reassuring warmth of this amber concoction.

*Recipe:*Lemon-Basil Quinoa Salad:

Components:

- One cup of chilled, cooked quinoa

- Half a cup of cherry tomatoes

- Half a cup diced cucumber

- 1/4 cup coarsely chopped red onion

- Finely chopped fresh basil leaves

Getting dressed:

- Three teaspoons pure olive oil

- One lemon, juiced and zest

- One teaspoon of oregano, dried

- Season with salt and pepper to taste

Getting ready:

• Combine the quinoa, cucumber, red onion, cherry tomatoes, and basil in a big bowl.

• Combine olive oil, oregano, lemon zest, lemon juice, salt, and pepper in a small bowl.

• Drizzle the salad with the dressing and toss to fully incorporate.

• To let the flavours mingle, chill in the refrigerator for at least half an hour before serving.

Recipe: Spiced Sweet Potato Soup with Cumin:

Components:

- Two big sweet potatoes, chopped and skinned

- One chopped onion

- Three minced garlic cloves

- One teaspoon of cumin powder

- One-half tsp smoked paprika

- Four cups broth made with vegetables

- Season with salt and pepper to taste

- Fresh cilantro for decorating

Getting ready:

- Saute the onion and garlic in a big saucepan until they become tender.

• Stir to coat after adding the sweet potatoes, cumin, and smoky paprika.

• Add the veggie broth and heat until it boils. Once the sweet potatoes are soft, lower the heat and simmer them.

• Blend with an immersion blender until smooth. Add pepper and salt for seasoning.

• Before serving, garnish with fresh cilantro to give each mouthful a burst of freshness.

Recipe: **A Lentil Stew Infused with Rosemary:**

Components:

• One cup well-rinsed green or brown lentils

• Diced one onion

• Two sliced carrots

- Two sliced celery stalks

- Three minced garlic cloves

- One tsp of dehydrated rosemary

- Four cups broth made with vegetables

- One 14-ounce can of chopped tomatoes

- Season with salt and pepper to taste

Getting ready:

- Saute the onion, celery, carrots, and garlic in a big saucepan until they are tender.

- Add the diced tomatoes with their juice, lentils, rosemary, and vegetable broth.

- After bringing to a boil, lower the heat, and cook the lentils until they are soft.

- Adjust the flavours as required by adding salt and pepper to taste.

- Serve hot so that every mouthful is infused with the flavour of fragrant rosemary.

Recipe: **Cauliflower Roasted with Cinnamon and Turmeric:**

Components:

- One head of chopped cauliflower

- Two teaspoons of olive oil

- One tsp finely ground turmeric

- One tsp finely ground cinnamon

- Season with salt and pepper to taste

- As a garnish, fresh parsley

Getting ready:

Set the oven's temperature to 425°F (220°C).

- Combine the olive oil, turmeric, cinnamon, salt, and pepper in a bowl with the cauliflower florets.

- Arrange the cauliflower in a single layer on a baking pan.

- Roast for 25 to 30 minutes in the oven, or until crispy and golden brown.

- Before serving, garnish with fresh parsley to give this spicy meal a burst of freshness.

Final Thought: A Harmony of Restorative Tastes

"Fibromyalgia Vegan Delights" encourages you to revel in the anti-inflammatory herbs and spices' restorative symphony in Chapter 11. Every dish is proof of the incredible power that exists in your kitchen, a power that can both satisfy your taste and help you manage the symptoms of fibromyalgia while also promoting wellbeing. May you discover solace, peace, and a fresh understanding of the transformative power of nature's abundant supply of healing herbs as you embrace these fragrant wonders.

Chapter 12: Techniques for Effortless Meal Preparation

With the hectic pace of contemporary life and time being a valuable resource, Chapter 12 offers Meal Prep Strategies that are easy for people with fibromyalgia to incorporate into their daily routines. This chapter is not only about recipes; it's also about creating a kitchen haven that encourages convenience, effectiveness, and sustenance.

Recipe: **Make This Quinoa and Roasted Vegetable Bowl Once, Eat It Twice.**

Components:

• One cup raw quinoa

• A variety of veggies, such as cherry tomatoes, zucchini, and bell peppers

• To roast, mix olive oil, salt, and pepper.

• Hummus should be served

Getting ready:

- Prepare the quinoa per the directions on the box.

Start the oven to 400°F, or 200°C.

- Dice veggies into small pieces.

- Combine salt, pepper, and olive oil with the veggies.

- Roast until soft, 20 to 25 minutes.

- Spoon roasted veggies and cooked quinoa into meal containers.

When serving, add a dollop of hummus.

Tip: To provide a fast and wholesome base for dinners, roast a bigger quantity of veggies to use in different ways throughout the week.

Recipe: Happiness in a Buddha Bowl: Chickpea and Avocado Version

Components:

• One can (15 ounces) of rinsed and drained chickpeas

• One sliced avocado

• Greens mix (arugula, spinach and kale)

• Halved cherry tomatoes

• Tahini-lemon dressing

Getting ready:

• For 20 minutes, roast chickpeas at 400°F (200°C) in the oven.

To make the lemon-tahini dressing, combine tahini, olive oil, lemon juice, and salt.

- Spoon roasted chickpeas, cherry tomatoes, avocado slices, and mixed greens into meal containers.

- Just before serving, drizzle with the lemon-tahini dressing.

Advice: To keep the salad fresh, make the dressing separately and add it just before you eat.

Recipe: **A Taste of the Mediterranean: Stuffed Bell Peppers**

Components:

- Four bell peppers, any hue

- A cup of quinoa, cooked

- One can (15 ounces) of rinsed and drained chickpeas

- One cup of chopped cherry tomatoes

- Half a cup diced cucumber

- 1/4 cup coarsely chopped red onion

- Sliced Kalamata olives

- Hummus should be served

Getting ready:

- Set oven temperature to 375°F, or 190°C.

- Slice off the bell peppers' tops, then remove the seeds and membranes.

- Combine the cooked quinoa, chickpeas, cucumber, red onion, cherry tomatoes, and Kalamata olives in a bowl.

- Stuff the quinoa mixture into each bell pepper.

- Bake peppers for 25 to 30 minutes, or until they are soft.

Top with a generous portion of hummus.

For future easy and nutritious meals, freeze extra stuffed peppers after doubling the batch.

Recipe: Stir-fried Tofu Teriyaki: A Perfect Weekend Dinner

Components:

- One block of pressed and diced extra-firm tofu

- Vegetables in mixed stir-fries (broccoli, bell peppers, and snap peas)

- Sauce Teriyaki

- To serve, brown rice

Getting ready:

• In a pan, cook cubed tofu until golden brown.

• Tender-crisp mixed vegetables should be stir-fried.

• Cover the mixture with teriyaki sauce and return the tofu to the pan.

• Simmer for a further two to three minutes.

• Accompany with brown rice.

Advice: For best flavour, make extra teriyaki sauce, store it separately, and add it right before reheating.

Recipe: **Sheet Pan Fajita Bowl: An Easy One-Pan Wonder**

Components:

- One pound (450g) of sliced seitan or tofu

- Seasoning for fajitas

- Slicing bell peppers thinly

- A finely sliced red onion

- Tacos made with whole grains

Getting ready:

Start the oven to 400°F, or 200°C.

- Combine seitan or tofu with spice for fajitas.

- Arrange on a baking pan with the onions and peppers cut into slices.

- Give it a 20–25 minute roast.

- Accompany with tacos made from healthy grains.

Advice: Prepare additional fajita ingredients in bulk for simple assembly all week long.

Closure: Preparing Culinary Harmony in Ahead

When it comes to managing fibromyalgia, effective meal planning is the first step towards long-term health and wellbeing. With a symphony of flavours and textures provided in Chapter 12, people with fibromyalgia may enjoy healthy meals without having to worry about everyday cooking duties. Prepare once, enjoy twice, and set out on a gastronomic adventure where each mouthful contributes to healing, recovery, and well-being.

Chapter 13: Integration of a Holistic Lifestyle

The most important part of your culinary adventure is "Holistic Lifestyle Integration," where we explain how to include fibromyalgia-friendly vegan foods into your everyday routine. This chapter provides a manual for changing your lifestyle, accepting healthiness, and building resilience in the face of fibromyalgia—it's not only about cooking. Together, we will examine doable tactics, conscientious decisions, and delectable dishes that serve as pillars for healing, alleviation, and recovery.

1. Preparing Meals in Advance for Wellness

Proactive meal planning is the cornerstone of a healthy lifestyle. It's a plan that gives you the ability to make deliberate decisions, reduce stress, and make sure you have fibromyalgia-friendly items on hand all week. Let's look at a real-world illustration:

First example: Weekly Menu

Monday:

• Chickpea Avocado Salad Bowl for lunch

• Brown rice with lentil and vegetable curry for dinner

Wednesday

For a light lunch, try the Quinoa Berry Breakfast Bowl.

• Quinoa-stuffed peppers with roasted vegetables for dinner

This Friday:

• Snack-style lunch: Sweet Potato Hummus Bites

• Stir-fried savoury tempeh for dinner

This methodical technique guarantees diversity, nutritional equilibrium, and a blend of tastes, enhancing general well-being and managing fibromyalgia.

2. Effective Techniques for Grocery Shopping

A well-thought-out shopping list may help you navigate the grocery store more efficiently and with less overwhelm. Here's an example of vegan lifestyle that's suitable for those with fibromyalgia:

Example 2: A Grocery List Adapted to Fibromyalgia

• Fresh Vegetables:

• Leafy greens (kale, spinach)

- Vibrant veggies, such as cherry tomatoes and bell peppers

- Fresh herbs (cilantro, parsley)

- Proteins:

- Legumes (lentils, chickpeas)

- Proteins derived from plants (tofu, tempeh)

- Whole Grains:

- Brown rice and quinoa

- Good Fats:

- Nuts, avocado, and olive oil

- Dairy Substitutes:

Almond milk and plant-based yoghurt

- Herbs & Spices:

- Garlic, ginger, and turmeric

You will have everything you need for a week of vegan meals that are suitable for people with fibromyalgia thanks to this well chosen list.

3. Clever Meal Planning Methods

When it comes to treating fibromyalgia, efficiency is essential. Using clever meal prep strategies may greatly lessen the stress that comes with cooking every day. Let's look at a real-world illustration:

Recipe: **Roasted Vegetable Medley Prepared in Batch**

Components:

- A variety of veggies, including cherry tomatoes, bell peppers, and zucchini

- Sea salt, pepper, and olive oil

Getting ready:

Start the oven to 400°F, or 200°C.

- Dice veggies into small pieces.

- Combine salt, pepper, and olive oil.

- After spreading, roast for 20 to 25 minutes on a baking sheet.

- Let cool completely before dividing into servings.

Batch cooking like this gives a varied ingredient basis for many meals throughout the week, decreasing daily cooking labour.

4. Creating a Fibromyalgia-Friendly Kitchen Environment

Transforming your kitchen into a fibromyalgia-friendly paradise demands strategic organising and ergonomic considerations. Here's a realistic upgrade example:

Example 4: Fibromyalgia-Friendly Kitchen Upgrades

• Ergonomic Tools:

• Comfortable grip utensils to decrease strain.

• Adjustable-height chopping board for individual accessibility.

• Organizational Solutions:

• Clear containers for optimal ingredient sight.

• Frequently used objects at easy reach to reduce bending and reaching.

These additions increase your kitchen experience, making it a haven of comfort and delight.

5. Mindful Mealtime Rituals

Establishing mindful mealtime routines gives your daily schedule an additional degree of wellbeing. As an example, consider this:

Example 5: Evening Tea Ceremony - Mindful Mealtime Ritual

• Establish a Calm Space:

• For dining linens, use muted, calming hues.

• Put on some mellow background instrumental music.

• Make Mindful Food Choices:

- Savour each taste with little nibbles.

- Store electrical gadgets to reduce distractions.

You can make every mealtime an opportunity for self-care by bringing mindfulness into the process.

In conclusion, a holistic wellness blueprint

This chapter offers a roadmap for coping with fibromyalgia in the context of a comprehensive lifestyle integration. Each element supports a harmonious lifestyle, from proactive meal planning to effective grocery shopping, clever food prep methods, and designing a kitchen that is fibromyalgia-friendly. I hope that as you put these techniques into practice, you will find the support, happiness, and sustenance you need to overcome any obstacles that fibromyalgia may throw at you. Welcome to a life where taste and well-being coexist to create a haven of healing, solace, and recovery.

Chapter 14: Mild Movement and Exercise for Fibromyalgia

Movement becomes a song in the rhythmic dance of health and well-being, a healing symphony that reverberates through the body's corridors. A celebration of mild movement and exercise, Chapter 14 is designed especially for anyone navigating the complex terrain of fibromyalgia. Here, we not only discuss the advantages of mindful exercises like yoga and stretching, but we also provide nutritional foods to go along with these practices to enhance their overall health benefits.

Overview of the Holistic Movement

We discover a haven for body and mind in the soft embrace of movement. The first section of this chapter examines the many advantages of holistic movement, including how yoga and stretching may improve flexibility, reduce muscular stiffness, and improve the overall health of fibromyalgia sufferers.

Stretching and Yoga: A Pathway to Comfort

Example 1: Flow Yoga Morning Practice

Components:

• A cosy yoga mat

• Supporting cushions or bolsters

Getting ready:

• To begin, practise deep breathing. Sit comfortably and take slow, deep breaths, paying attention to each inhalation and exhalation.

• Gentle Neck Stretches: To relieve tension in your neck, gently tilt your head forward, backward, and side to side.

- Sun Salutations: To awaken the body and warm up the muscles, do a sequence of sun salutations.

- Seated positions: For grounding, try sitting positions like Padmasana (lotus pose) and Sukhasana (easy pose).

- Restorative positions: To conclude, do relaxing positions that promote healing, such as Child's Pose and Savasana.

Remember to pay attention to your body and adjust positions as necessary, prioritising comfort above intensity.

Recipes that Go Along with Movement

For the best possible performance and recuperation after mild activity, make sure your body is well nourished before and after. This section offers dishes to go along with your yoga or stretching practice that are made using ingredients that are suitable to fibromyalgia sufferers.

Recipe: Boosting Smoothie Before Yoga

Components:

• One mature banana

• One-half cup berries (strawberries, blueberries)

• One-third cup chia seeds

• One cup of spinach leaves

• One cup almond milk

Getting ready:

• Blend All Ingredients: In a blender, combine almond milk, spinach, chia seeds, bananas, and berries.

• Blend Until Smooth: Continue blending until a smooth consistency is reached.

• Pour and Savour: For long-lasting energy, pour this nutrient-rich smoothie into a glass and enjoy 30 minutes before your yoga practice.

Recipe: **Protein Balls After Workout**

Components:

• One cup of rolled oats

• Half a cup of almond or peanut butter

• One-fourth cup maple syrup

• Grounded flaxseed, half a cup

• Half a cup of protein powder that is vegan

• One tsp vanilla essence

Getting ready:

- Combine Dry Ingredients: In a dish, mix vegan protein powder, powdered flaxseed, and rolled oats.

- Add Wet Ingredients: Mix in vanilla essence, maple syrup, and nut butter.

- Form Balls: Roll the ingredients into bite-sized balls using your palms.

- Chill: To set, place the protein balls in the fridge for a minimum of half an hour.

- Savour: After your exercise, grab a few protein balls for a tasty and high-protein snack.

A Guided Stretching Programme for the Relief of Fibromyalgia

Example 4: Stretching routine in the evening

Components:

• A cosy area equipped with a yoga mat

• Props for support, such as pillows or cushions

Getting ready:

• Shoulder and Neck Stretch: To relieve tension in your shoulders and neck, gently slant your head from side to side.

• Back Stretch: While sitting with your legs crossed on the mat, extend your back by reaching forward.

• Seated Twist: To strengthen your core and lengthen your spine, gently twist from side to side.

Leg stretches: To lengthen your hamstrings, extend your legs and reach for your toes.

• Child's Pose: Unwind in this pose that stretches your hips and lower back.

Note: To improve relaxation, move slowly and deliberately, holding each stretch for 15 to 30 seconds while concentrating on taking deep breaths.

Snack After Stretching for Recuperation

Muscle rehabilitation requires proper post-stretching body support. This area offers a quick and healthy snack to help you feel reenergized.

Recipe: **Nut-Berry Parfait**

Components:

• One cup of mixed berries (blueberries and strawberries)

- Half a cup of vegan yoghurt

- One-fourth cup granola

- 1 tablespoon of finely chopped nuts (walnuts, almonds)

Getting ready:

- Layering Ingredients: Arrange chopped nuts, granola, mixed berries, and vegan yoghurt in a glass.

- Continue stacking: Continue stacking until you get to the top of the glass.

- Present and Savour: Indulge in this delicious parfait, relishing the blend of flavours and textures.

In summary, a comprehensive dance of well-being

In Chapter 14, you're invited to join the elegant dance of low-impact exercise and movement, using recipes that improve your body's health and well-being. May every stretch, breath, and bite become a harmonic expression of self-care and renewal as you explore the carefully chosen routines and savour the fibromyalgia-friendly treats. Accept the holistic dance of health and allow it to serve as your road map to recovery, alleviation, and a happier, healthier existence.

Chapter 15: Integration of a Holistic Lifestyle

In the grand conclusion of 'Fibromyalgia Vegan Delights', we dive into the practice of integrating a holistic lifestyle and turn the cookbook into a thorough manual for incorporating vegan meals that are good for fibromyalgia into everyday life. This chapter offers a guide for cultivating a well-rounded, conscious, and nutritious life rather than just a list of recipes.

1. Harmonising Diet, Exercise, and Mindfulness: A Wellness Symphony

Introduction: We examine the trinity of exercise, mindfulness, and nutrition in the search for holistic well-being. People with fibromyalgia may develop a lifestyle that goes beyond the kitchen and encompasses all aspects of their everyday routine by balancing these components.

Example 1: A Conscious Morning Schedule:

• Morning Meditation: To establish a pleasant attitude for the day, begin with a five-minute mindfulness meditation.

• Stretching Routine: To enhance flexibility and arouse the body, do light stretches.

2. Mindful Eating Environment Creation: Fostering Happy Mealtimes

Introduction: Eating mindfully involves more than just the items on your plate. It's about embracing the journey of food from farm to table, relishing each mouthful, and setting up a setting that makes mealtimes joyful.

Example 2: A tranquil eating area

• Select Calm Colours: Use blues and greens to create a relaxing atmosphere in your dining room.

- Soft Lighting: To create a cosy ambiance, use warm, soft lighting.

- Calm Ambient Noises: During meals, play soft instrumental music or natural noises.

3. Nutrition and Taste Harmony: The Foundation of Every Recipe

Introduction: The goal of every dish in this chapter is to achieve nutritional balance while stimulating the senses of taste. We investigate recipes that embrace flavour richness and provide a range of nutrients.

Recipe: **Quinoa Berry Breakfast Bowl, for instance:**

- Components:

- A cup of quinoa, cooked

- Strawberries, blueberries, and raspberries are mixed berries.

- Drizzle of almond butter

- Chia seeds as a garnish

Getting ready:

- As the foundation, arrange cooked quinoa in a bowl.

- Add a colourful mixture of berries on top.

- For extra richness, drizzle almond butter over.

- Add chia seeds as a garnish to increase the nutritional value.

4. Calm Movement and Exercise: Taking Care of the Body

Introduction: Recognising the special requirements of people with fibromyalgia, we provide easy motions and exercises that improve general health without putting unnecessary pressure on the body.

Example 4: Doing Yoga to Unwind

• Order:

• Start by practicing deep breathing.

• Mild rotations and strains of the neck.

• Forward bends while seated for flexibility.

Conclude with a peaceful meditation.

**5. Conscientious Meal Planning: A Tactician's Guide to Success in the Kitchen

Introduction: Taking a deliberate approach to meal planning turns it into an art. We provide advice on creating a diet plan that promotes general health and complies with fibromyalgia-friendly guidelines.

Example No. 5: Weekly Menu:

• Day 1: Steamed asparagus with baked lemon herb tilapia for dinner, followed by a quinoa and berry breakfast bowl and a chickpea and avocado salad bowl.

• Day 3: Brown rice with lentil and vegetable curry for supper and sweet potato hummus bites for snack.

• Dinner on Day 5 is Grilled Tofu Skewers with Quinoa Pilaf.

**6. Using Anti-Inflammatory Herbs and Spices for Holistic Healing

Introduction: Explore the world of therapeutic spices and herbs that may help control the symptoms of fibromyalgia. The characteristics of important components are discussed in this part along with ways to include them in your regular diet.

Recipe: Golden Milk with Ginger and Turmeric

• Components:

• One cup plant-based milk (coconut or almond).

• Half a teaspoon of turmeric powder

• One-fourth teaspoon of ground ginger

• A dash of cayenne

• To taste, sweetener (agave, maple syrup)

Getting ready:

• In a saucepan, warm the plant-based milk.

- Include the ginger, turmeric, and black pepper.

Stir well and cook for five minutes.

- For a calming effect, sweeten to taste and eat just before bed.

In conclusion, a happy and nourishing lifestyle

In the latter chapters of "Fibromyalgia Vegan Delights," we encourage you to adopt these habits as the foundation of a lifestyle designed for healing, comfort, and recovery, rather than just as extras to your daily regimen. Every dish, mindful practice, and well-thought-out meal plan adds to a harmonious whole, offering sustenance, happiness, and the delicious flavours of vigorous living. I hope this chapter will serve as a roadmap, a friend, and a source of inspiration for you as you pursue a more vibrant and well-balanced life.

BONUS: MEAL PLANNER

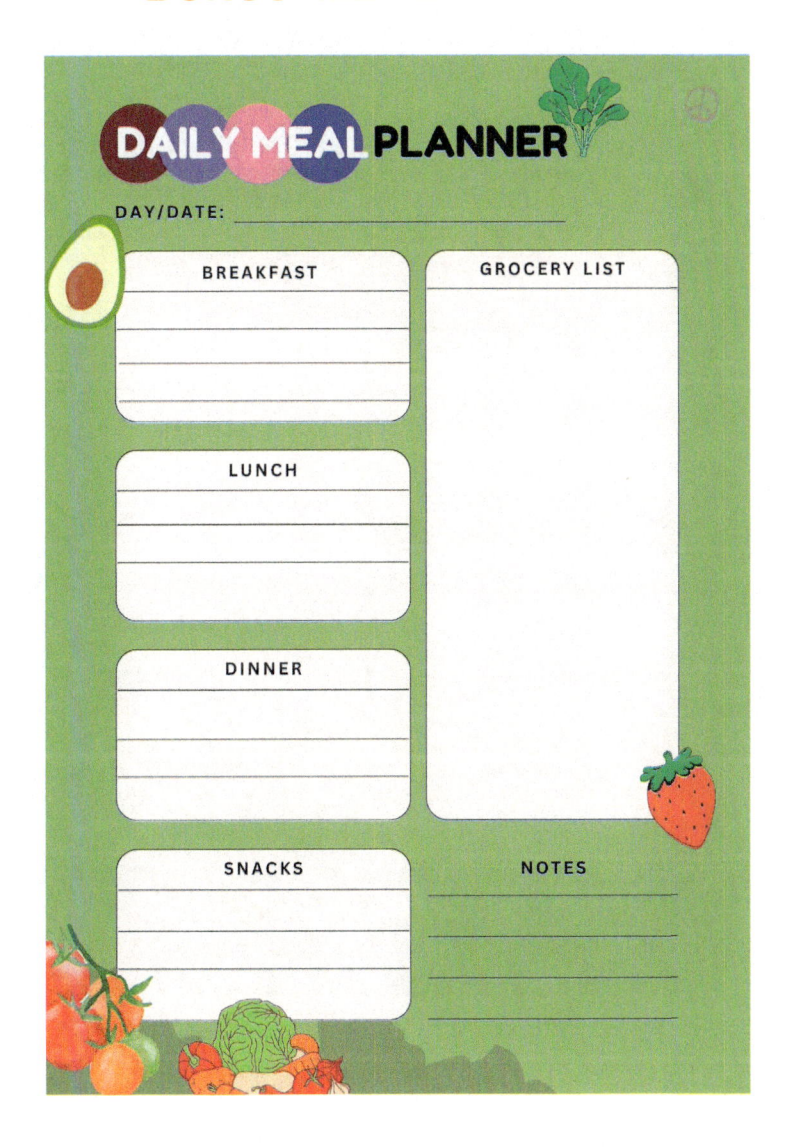

DAILY MEAL PLANNER

DAY/DATE: _____

BREAKFAST

LUNCH

DINNER

SNACKS

GROCERY LIST

NOTES

DAILY MEAL PLANNER

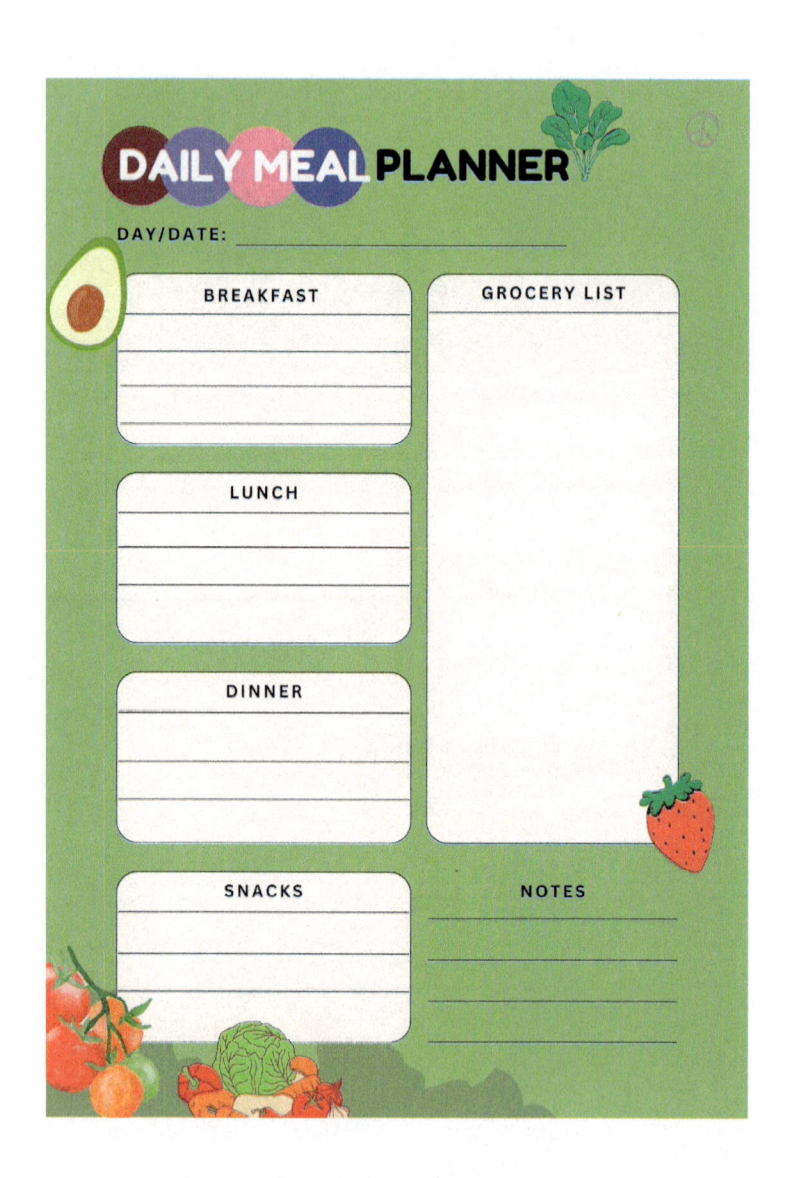

DAY/DATE: _____

BREAKFAST

LUNCH

DINNER

SNACKS

GROCERY LIST

NOTES

DAILY MEAL PLANNER

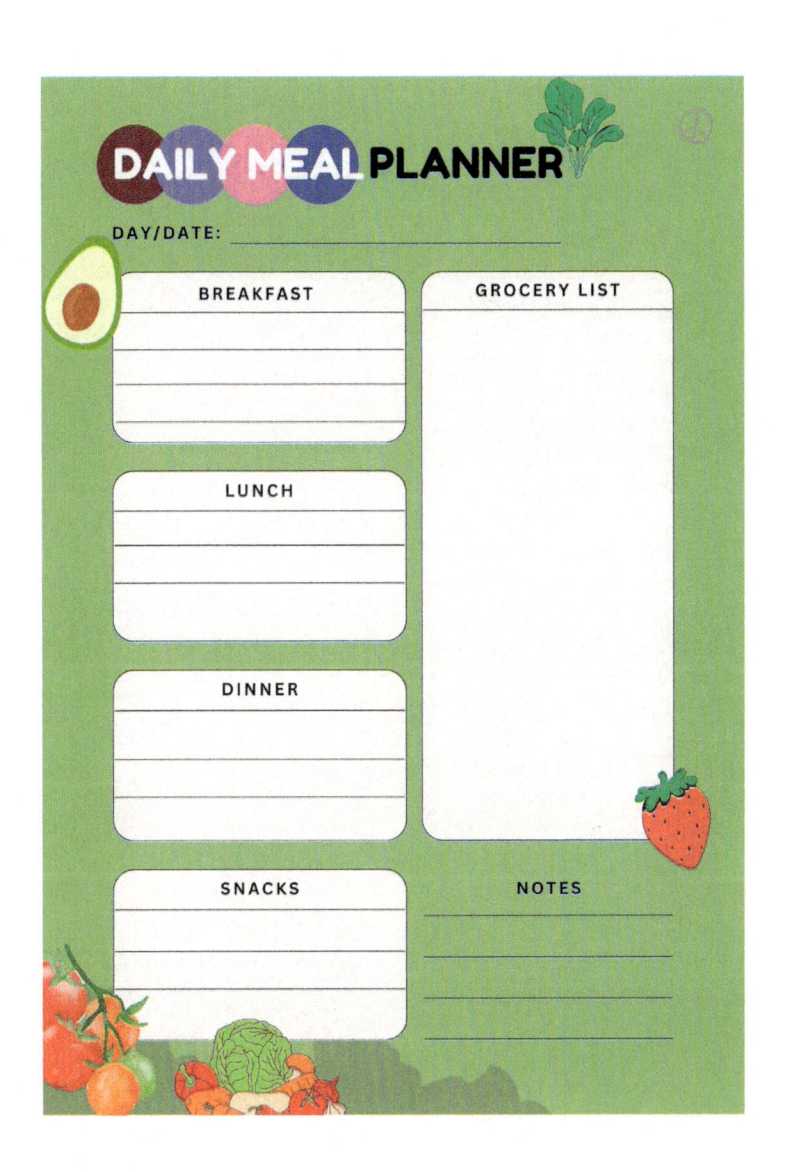

DAY/DATE: _____

BREAKFAST

LUNCH

DINNER

SNACKS

GROCERY LIST

NOTES

DAILY MEAL PLANNER

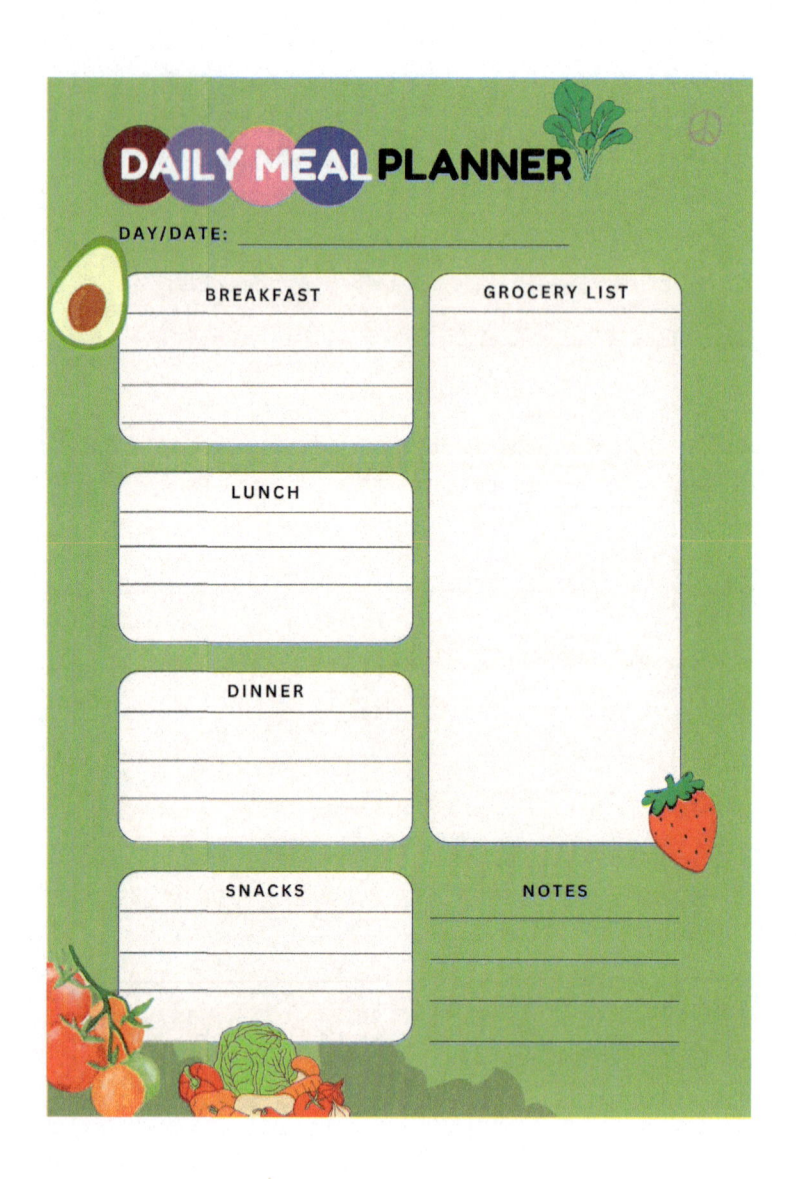

DAY/DATE: _____

BREAKFAST

LUNCH

DINNER

SNACKS

GROCERY LIST

NOTES

DAILY MEAL PLANNER

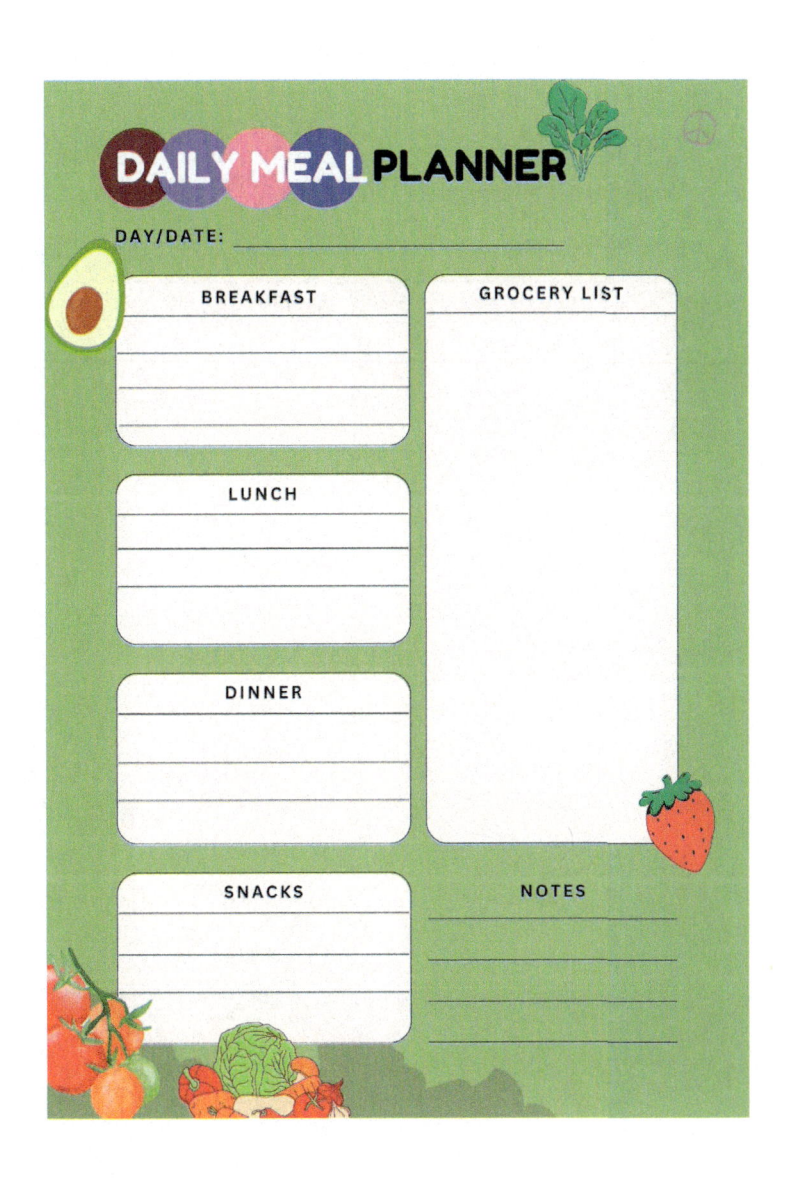

DAY/DATE: _____

BREAKFAST

LUNCH

DINNER

SNACKS

GROCERY LIST

NOTES

DAILY MEAL PLANNER

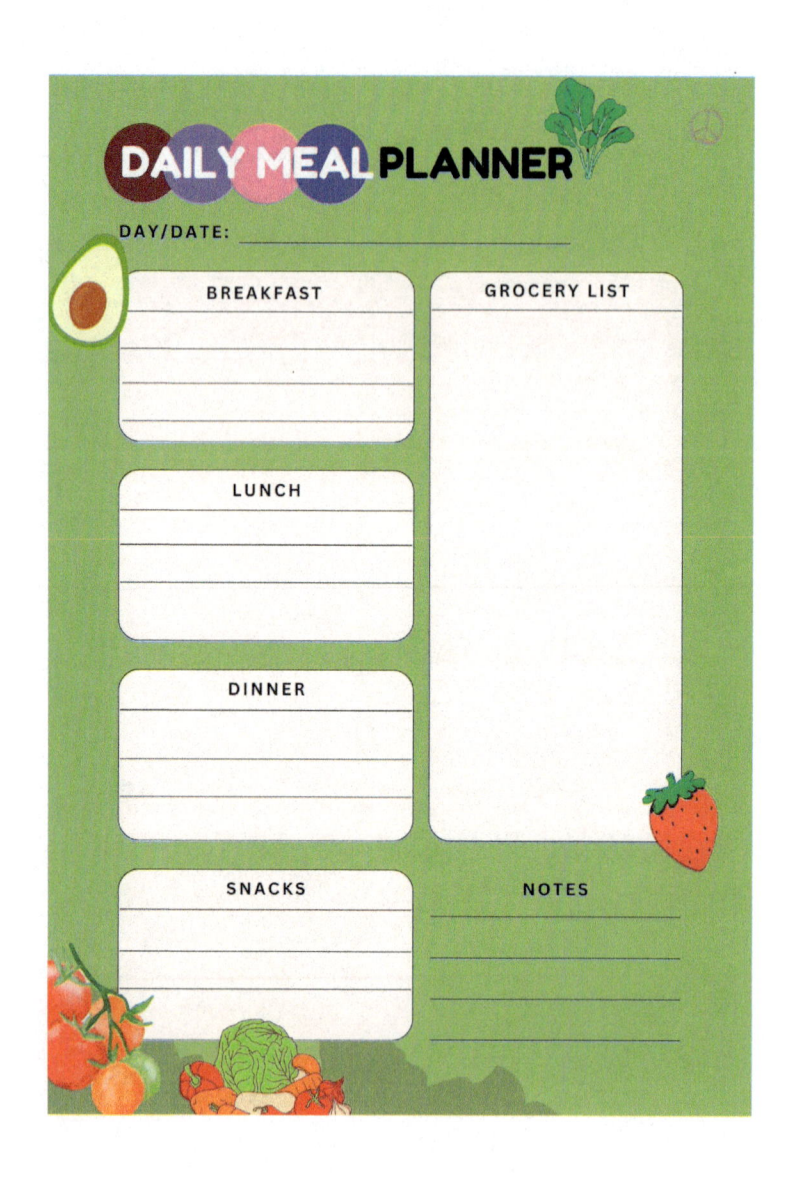

DAY/DATE: _____

BREAKFAST

LUNCH

DINNER

SNACKS

GROCERY LIST

NOTES

DAILY MEAL PLANNER

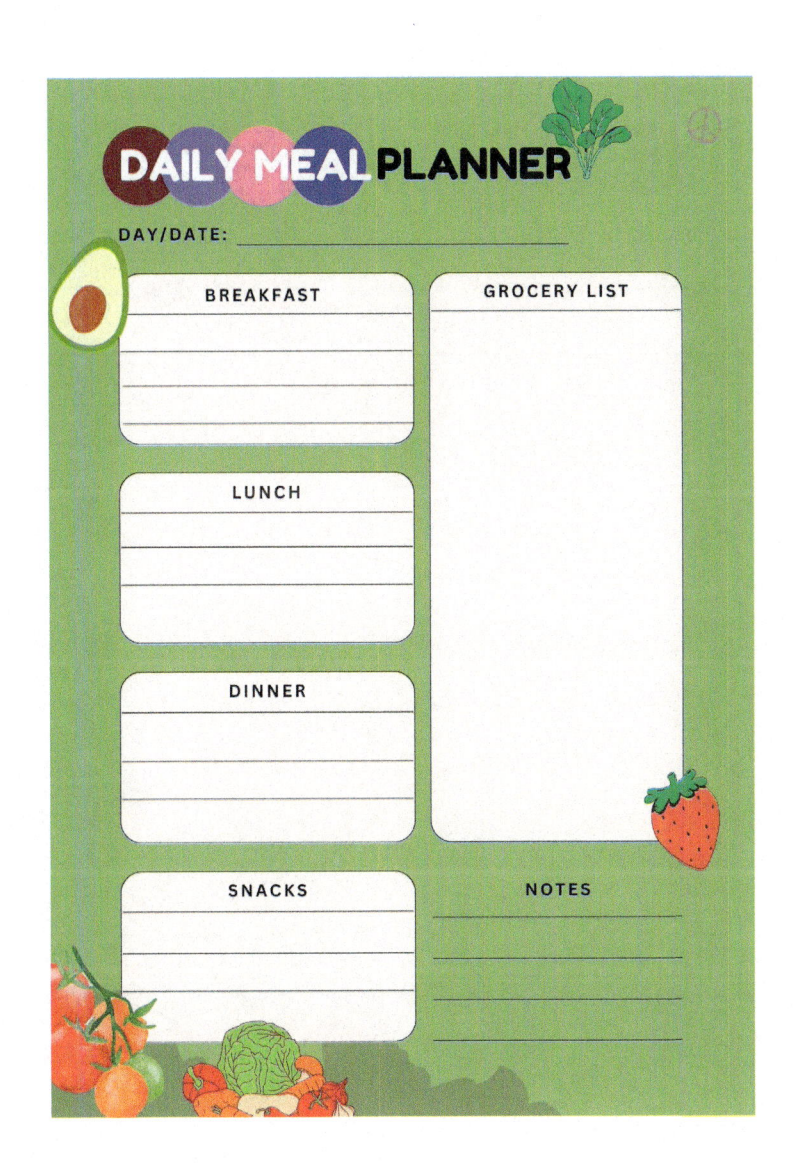

DAY/DATE: _____

BREAKFAST

LUNCH

DINNER

SNACKS

GROCERY LIST

NOTES

DAILY MEAL PLANNER

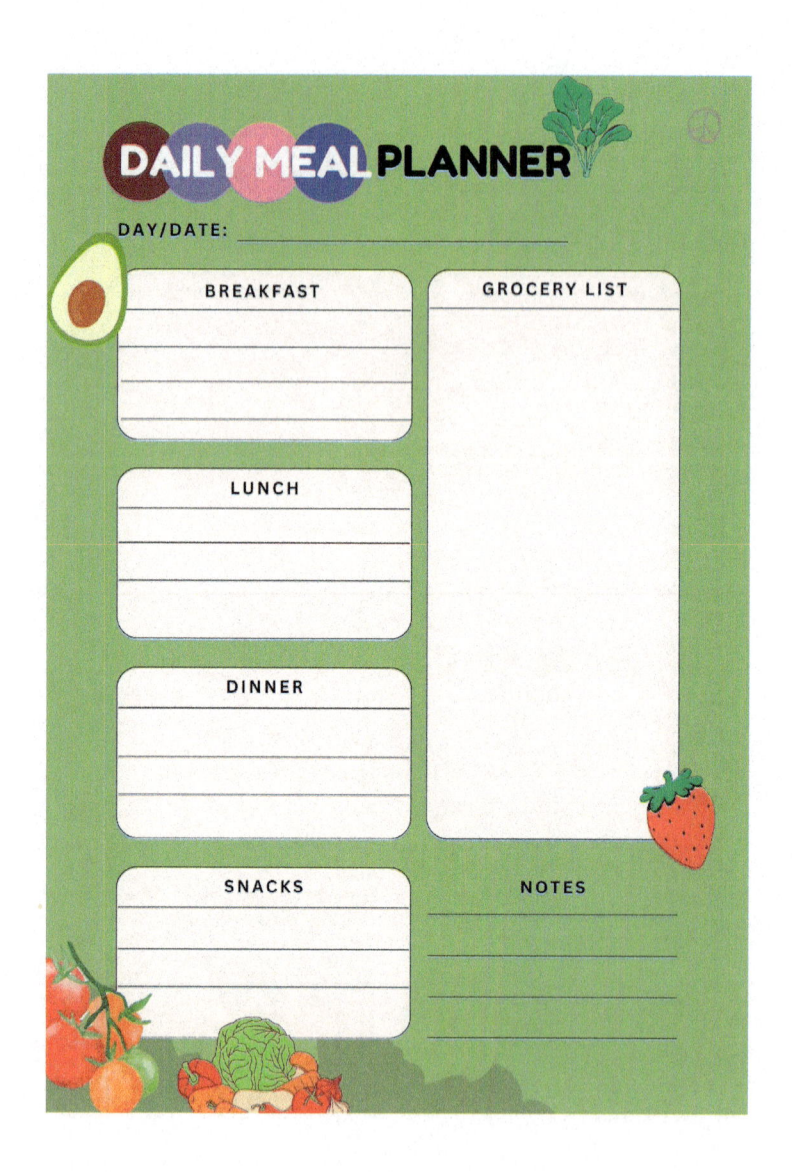

DAY/DATE: _____

BREAKFAST

LUNCH

DINNER

SNACKS

GROCERY LIST

NOTES

DAILY MEAL PLANNER

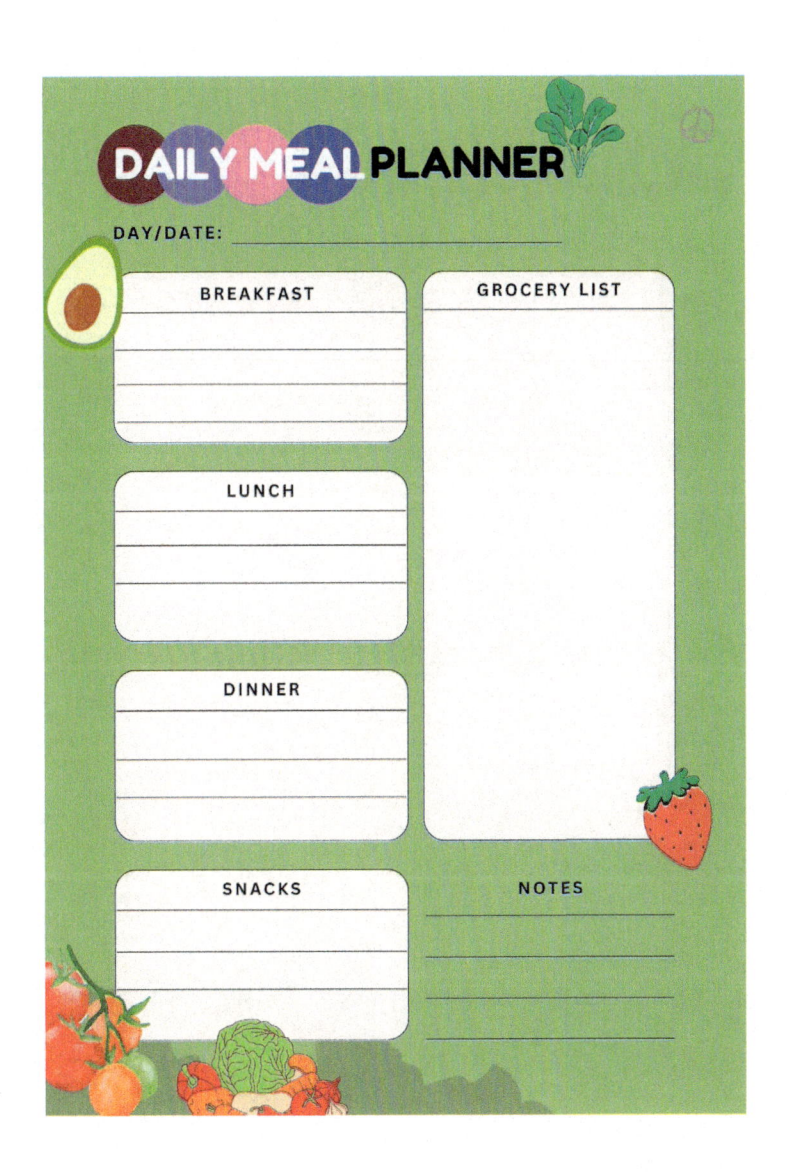

DAY/DATE: _____

BREAKFAST

LUNCH

DINNER

SNACKS

GROCERY LIST

NOTES

DAILY MEAL PLANNER

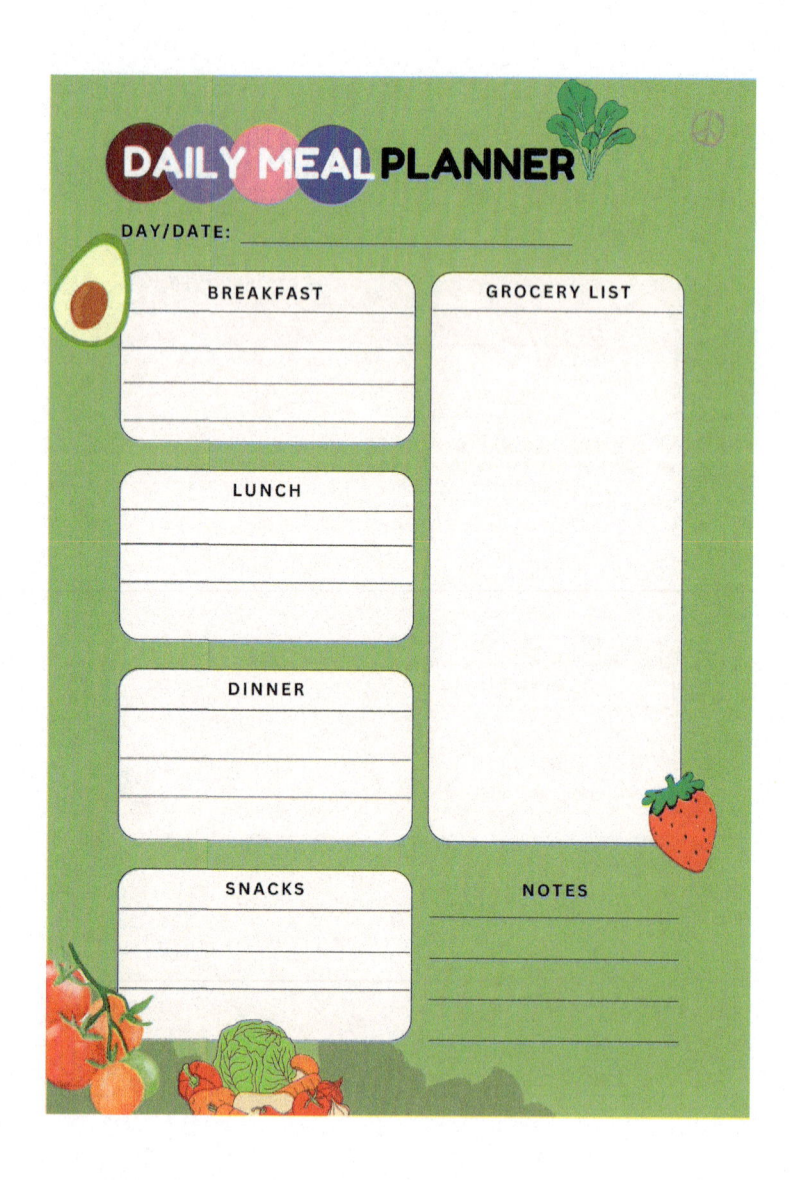

DAY/DATE: _____

BREAKFAST

LUNCH

DINNER

SNACKS

GROCERY LIST

NOTES

DAILY MEAL PLANNER

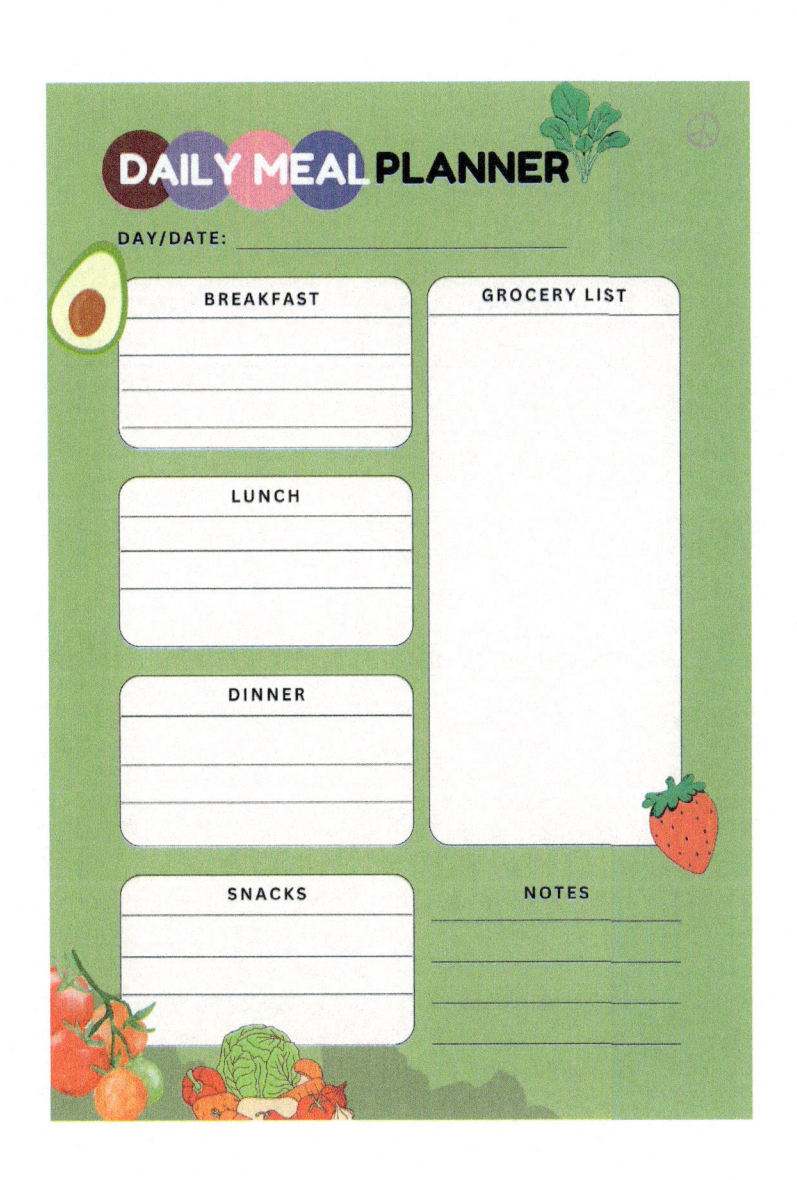

DAY/DATE: _____

BREAKFAST

LUNCH

DINNER

SNACKS

GROCERY LIST

NOTES

DAILY MEAL PLANNER

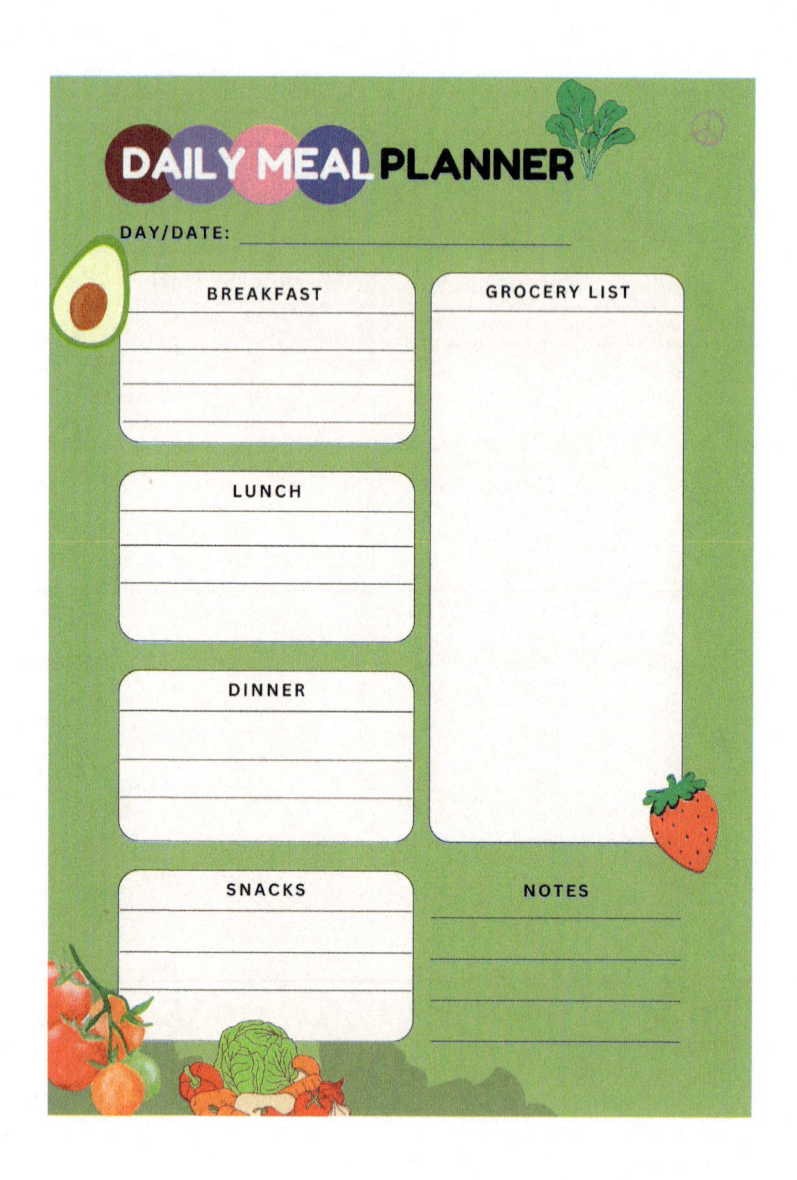

DAY/DATE: _____

BREAKFAST

LUNCH

DINNER

SNACKS

GROCERY LIST

NOTES

DAILY MEAL PLANNER

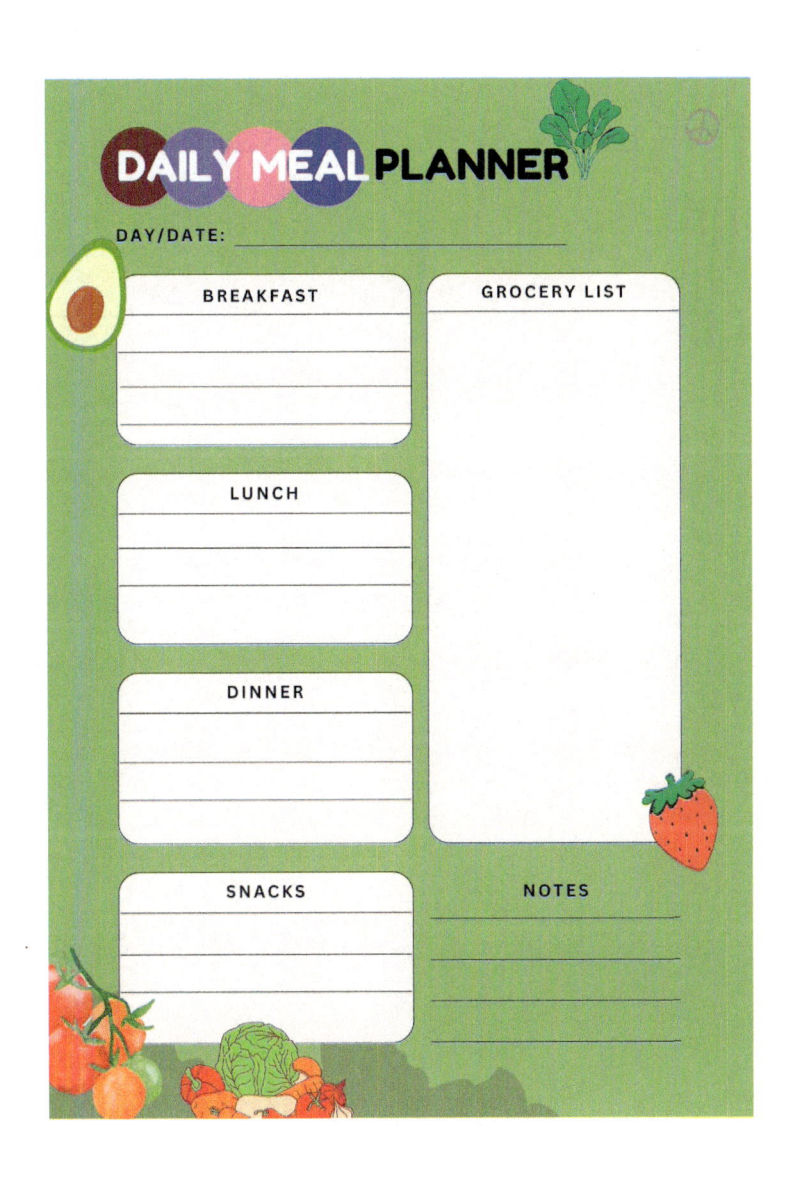

DAY/DATE: _____

BREAKFAST

LUNCH

DINNER

SNACKS

GROCERY LIST

NOTES

Printed in Great Britain
by Amazon